The Whole-Body Reset

A WAY OF EATING FOR THE REST OF YOUR LIFE

300 RECIPES,

100 DAYS OF MEAL PLAN

and MORNING EXERCISES

at MIDLIFE AND BEYOND

jonathan price

j o n a t h a n   p r i c e is an independent publisher, if you enjoy this book, please consider supporting us by leaving a review!

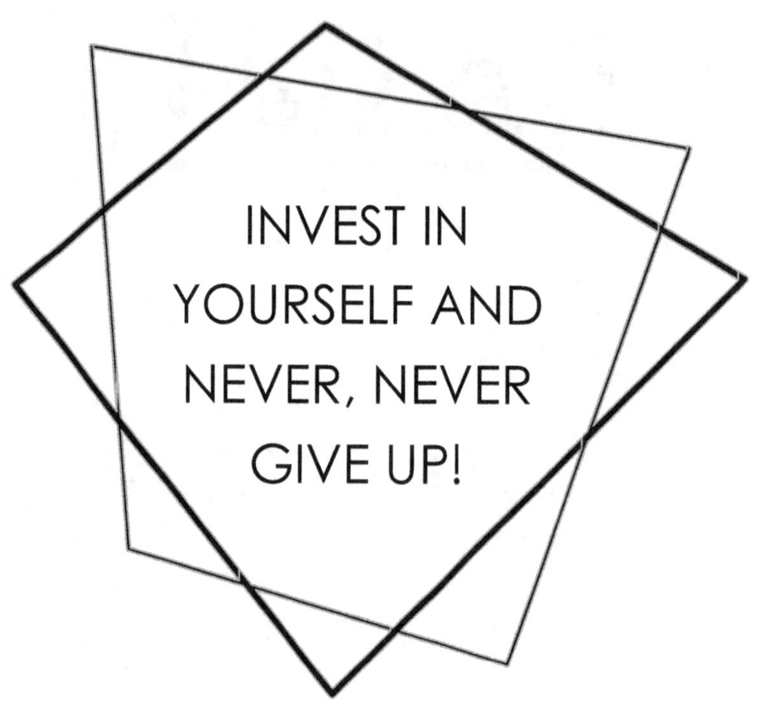

This book is designed to help you create a healthy and sustainable lifestyle. This book contains a 100-DAY MEAL PLAN. Each day includes **breakfast, lunch, and dinner**. The recipes are easy to follow and can be adapted to your preferences.

This book also contains MORNING EXERCISES that you can do to get your day started on the right foot. These routines are designed for adults over 50 years and can be modified to your fitness level.

If you're looking to reset your whole body, then this book is for you! For 100 days, you'll follow a meal plan with 300 RECIPES that will help you detox and rejuvenate your body. With food options for every taste, you'll be sure to find something that satisfies you. So get started on your journey to a new you today!

Contents

INTRODUCTION

The standard American diet is high in processed foods, refined carbs, and unhealthy fats. This way of eating can lead to various health problems, including obesity, type 2 diabetes, heart disease, and cancer.

Fortunately, there is a way to change all that. The whole-body reset is a comprehensive approach to eating that emphasizes whole, unprocessed foods, healthy fats, and moderate amounts of protein. This way of eating has been shown to improve health and help prevent chronic disease.

This book aims to help you get your day started on the right foot, make you feel more energetic and motivated, and improve your overall health. The whole-body reset is based on the premise that many chronic health problems in adults over 50 are caused by inflammation. Inflammation is the body's natural response to injury or infection. Still, when it becomes chronic, it can lead to a host of health problems such as heart disease, arthritis, diabetes, and cancer.

Body reset aims to reduce inflammation by eating a healthy diet and exercising regularly. It can be difficult to know how to start the day off right when you're in the midst of midlife. You may feel like you've been doing the same things for years and don't know where to begin. That's why we've created this 100- day meal plan and morning exercise routine! These activities will help start your day on the right foot and make you feel more energetic and motivated.

This is not a fad diet; it's a way of eating for the rest of your life. By following this plan, you'll improve your health and also feel better than you have in years.

ALLOWED FOODS & CONDIMENTS LIST

There are many foods and condiments that you can enjoy while following this meal plan. Here is a list of some of the items that are allowed:

- Fruits: apples, oranges, bananas, grapes, strawberries, watermelon, etc.
- Vegetables: carrots, celery, broccoli, spinach, kale, tomatoes, etc.
- Protein sources: chicken, fish, tofu, legumes, eggs, etc.
- Whole grains: quinoa, oats, brown rice, whole wheat bread, etc.
- Healthy fats: avocado, olive oil, nuts, seeds, etc.
- Herbs and spices: basil, oregano, pepper, garlic, ginger, etc.

FOODS TO AVOID

There are also some foods that you should avoid while following this meal plan. These items can sabotage your efforts to eat healthily and feel your best. Avoid these items:

- Refined grains: white bread, white rice, pastries, etc.
- Sugary drinks: soda, processed fruit juice, sports drinks, etc

- Added sugars: candy, cookies, cake, etc.
- Unhealthy fats: fried foods, margarine, shortening, etc.
- Artificial
  Ingredients: trans fats, Monosodium glutamate (MSG), food coloring, etc.

HOW TO USE THIS BOOK

Whole body resets are popular these days, and for a good reason. They can be extremely beneficial for your health, helping to improve everything from energy levels and digestion to sleep quality and immunity.

But if you're new to the world of whole-body resets, they can also seem a bit daunting. How exactly do you go about resetting within 100 days?

Here's a quick guide to get you started:

1. Start with a clean slate.

Before you begin your whole body reset, it's important to start with a clean slate. This means eliminating all processed foods, sugary drinks, and unhealthy habits from your life. If you're unsure where to start, try cutting out all processed foods and refined sugars for 21 days. This will help jumpstart your reset and give you a better sense of healthy eating.

2. Incorporate more whole foods into your diet.

Once you've eliminated processed foods and refined sugars from your diet, it's time to start incorporating more whole foods. This includes plenty of fruits and vegetables and healthy proteins and fats. Aim to fill your plate with at least half fruits and vegetables at every meal, and make sure to include a source of protein with each meal as well.

3. Drink plenty of water.

Staying hydrated is crucial for any reset, but it's especially important when trying to reset your whole body. Make sure to drink plenty of water throughout the day, and consider adding some lemon or lime wedges to your water for an extra boost of flavor.

4. Get moving.

Incorporating some form of exercise into your daily routine is a great way to help reset your body. It doesn't have to be too strenuous - even a simple walk around the block will do. Just make sure to get moving every day, and you'll see some results.

5. Reduce stress levels.

Stress can majorly impact your overall health, so it's important to find ways to reduce it when you're resetting your body. There are several ways to do this, but some simple things include getting regular exercise, practicing meditation or deep breathing, and spending time in nature.

By following these simple steps, you'll be well on your way to reset your whole body within 100 days. Just remember to be patient and take it.

MORNING EXERCISES

ALTERNATE NOSTRIL BREATHING (NADI SHODHANA)

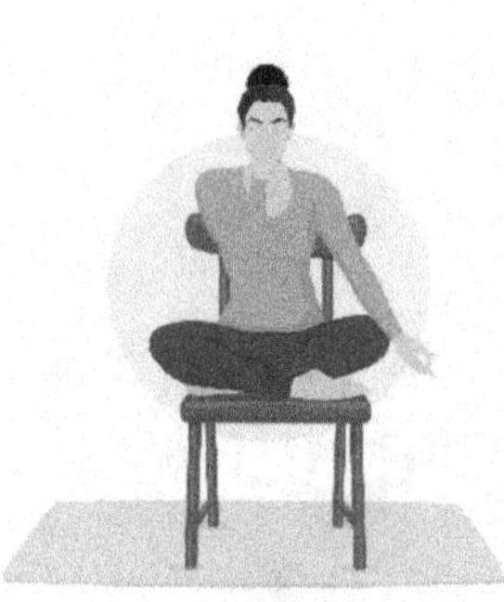

Paying attention to your breath quality and tracking its flow through your nostrils is one of the fastest ways to collect and calm yourself. This breathing technique calms you down immediately whenever you feel anxious or agitated. It also improves sleep and nasal respiration and boosts thinking.

Step-by-Step Instructions

- Sit up tall and comfortable in the chair with your spine erect and relaxed, feet planted firmly on the floor at about hip-width apart, and breathe in and out slowly through both nostrils to make yourself more comfortable.
- Place your right thumb on your right nostril and your ring finger or right forefinger on the left nostril maintaining light contact with them throughout. Close your right nostril by pressing it gently with the thumb and inhale through the left nostril.
- Release your thumb and close your left nostril by gently pressing it with your right forefinger or ring finger and breathe out through your left nostril.
- Repeat alternating between your left and right nostrils.

OCEAN BREATH (UJJAYI PRANAYAMA)

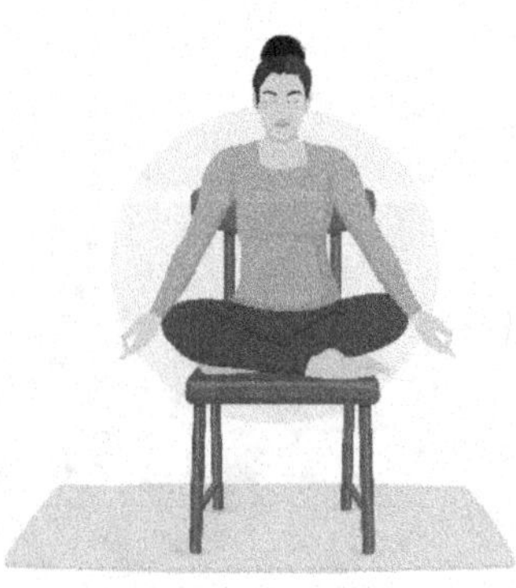

This yoga breathing technique is used when flowing and holding through postures. It helps you stay alert, relaxed, and energized.

Step-by-Step Instructions

- Sit up tall and comfortable in the chair with your feet flat on the ground.
- Rest your hands on your knees with palms facing upwards and thumbs and forefingers interlaced.
- Breathe in slightly deeper than normal through your nose, then breathe out with your mouth open and make a silent extended "haaaaah" sound. Repeat this twice.
- Now try to make a similar sound on both the inhalation and exhalation with your mouth closed and breathing through the nose. To achieve this, you will need to constrict your throat gently, closing off its back as you inhale.

CLEANSING BREATH (KAPALBHATI)

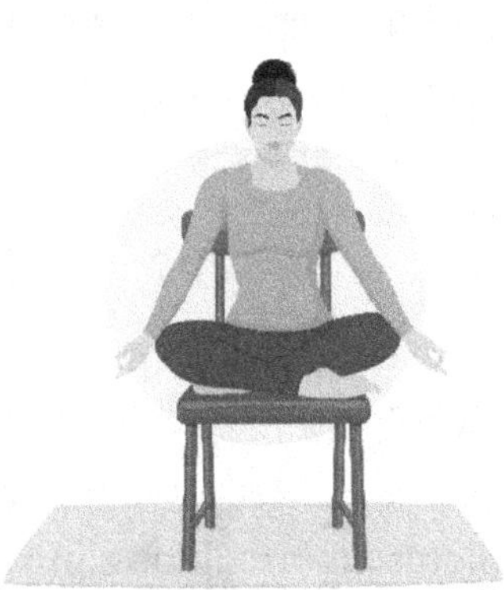

Kapalbhati Pranayama also known as "Skull Shining" is a famous yoga breathing technique among yogis for clearing the mind. This breathing technique is an excellent way to remove "cobwebs" in your mind and lungs and increase your concentration level. Besides, it helps work your core and lower abs, relieve stress, increase metabolism and boost energy.

Step-by-Step Instructions
- Sit up tall in the chair leaving some space behind you so that you are not leaning on it.
- Plant your feet flat and firmly on the floor with your hands hanging by your sides
- Rest your hands on your thighs just above the knees with palms facing up.
- Take a deep full breath in through your nose, then breathe out all the air as you pull your navel and the belly back towards the spine. Next, take a partial breath in and exhale quickly through the nose relaxing the navel and the abdomen. You may pump at a pace of your choice. Just ensure that the breath is continuous but the "breathe ins" are very subtle and small. Perform as many pumps as you can. Start smaller and build your way up.
- On the last pump, stop and take a full breath in and a full breath out.

BELLOWS BREATH (BHASTRIKA)

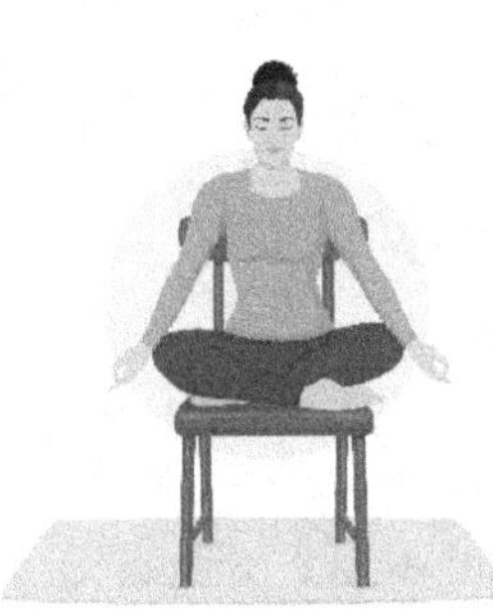

This type of yogic breathing helps energize and awaken your entire body. It also helps clear your mind, relieves stress from the brain, builds abdominal strength, increases your lung capacity, boosts digestion, and increases metabolism.

Step-by-Step Instructions
- Sit up tall in the chair with your hips towards the edge of the chair, back straight, your feet planted firmly on the floor at a hip-width apart.
- Place one hand on your belly and keep the other one resting on your thigh.
- Take a short forceful breath in followed by a short, sharp breath out.
- Do it over and over again for about one minute
- On the last pump, take a break before you repeat the pumping

BREATH RETENTION (KUMBHAKA)

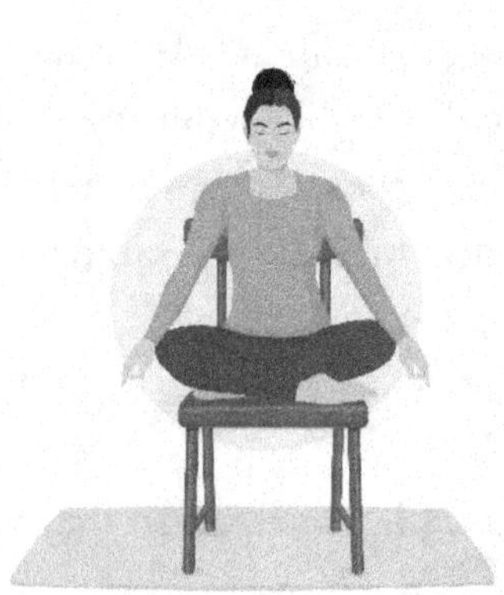

Just as the name suggests, Kumbhaka Pranayama is a breathing technique that involves holding the breath after inhaling or exhaling. Breath retention helps increase pressure in your lungs giving them time to fully expand, increasing their capacity. This increases the flow of oxygenated blood to the heart, brain, and muscles.

Step-by-Step Instructions
- Sit up tall in the chair with your hips towards the edge of the chair, back straight, your feet planted firmly on the floor at a hip-width apart.
- Take a deep, full breath in and try to picture it circulating in your heart. Lower your head down bringing your chin close to your chest as you inflate your lungs. Hold your breath until you feel you can no longer do it, then exhale all the air out.
- Once all the air is completely out, hold empty for as long as you can before inflating your lungs again.

COOLING BREATH (SITALI)

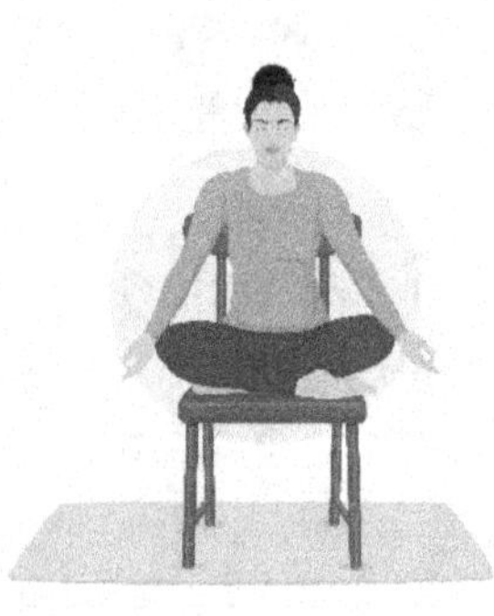

Sithali helps cool down and calm your body. Our bodies may become overheated due to changes in our external and internal temperatures, or after performing a yoga session or any other workout. Practicing this breathing technique will help you cool down when you feel overheated.

Step-by-Step Instruction
- Sit up tall in the chair with your hips towards the edge of the chair, back straight, your feet planted firmly on the floor at a hip-width apart.
- Place your palms face-down on your thighs.
- Take deep breaths in and out twice or thrice through your nose to prepare for this pranayama.
- Curl the sides of your tongue inwards towards the center to roll it into a tube-like shape. If you can't roll your tongue, purse your lips to make a small "o" shape with your mouth.
- Inhale slowly through the tube if you roll your tongue or channel the air through the "o" shaped opening if your lips are pursed.
- Close your mouth and breathe out slowly through your nose.
- Repeat until you feel the maximum cooling effect

HISSING TEETH BREATH (SITKARI)

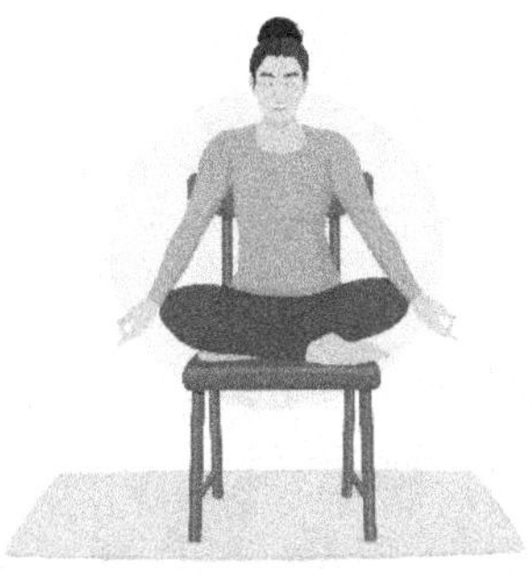

This is also another cooling breath technique that helps refresh the body and mind.

Step-by-Step Instruction

- Sit up tall in the chair with your hips towards the edge of the chair, back straight, your feet planted firmly on the floor at a hip-width apart.
- Take a few natural breaths in and out to center yourself.
- With your lips open, close your teeth by bringing your lower and upper teeth together and inhale through them producing a soft hissing sound.
- Release the teeth and close your mouth as you breathe out through the nose
- Repeat until you feel a nice cooling effect that eases your body and mind.

CHAIR MOUNTAIN POSE (CHAIR TADASANA)

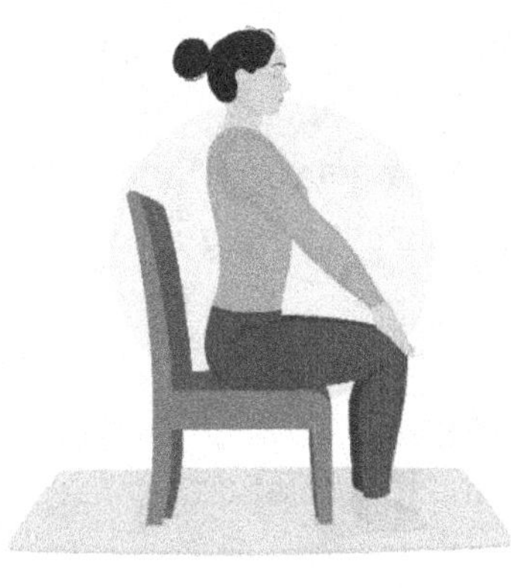

This chair yoga warm-up exercise helps calm your body and mind, making you feel more grounded and ready to perform other sequences. It warms up your back muscles, heart, and shoulder muscles.

Step-by-Step Instruction

- Begin by sitting up tall in your chair, leaving some space behind you.
- Keep your spine lengthened, shoulders neutral with chest raised, and engage your abdominal muscles.
- Plant your feet flat and firmly on the floor at a hip distance apart with toes pointed straight ahead.
- Keep your limbs and face relaxed
- Place your palms flat on top of your upper thighs
- Close your eyes and take 10-15 complete deep breaths in and out through your nose.
- Slowly and gently open your eyes and release your hands down by your sides to come out of the pose.

SEATED NECK ROLLS (KANTASANCHALANA)

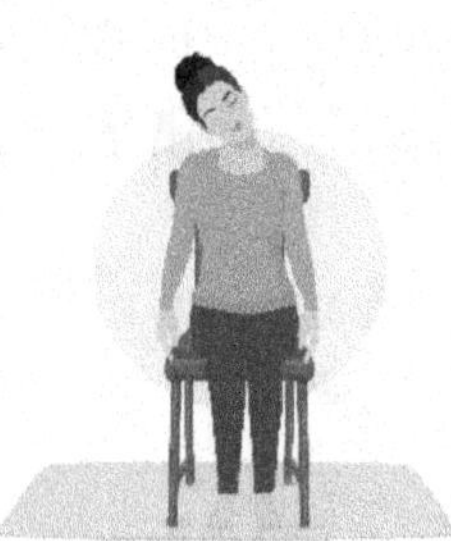

If you spend a lot of time sitting, neck rolls are the best warm-up for your chair yoga sequences. It helps release tension from your neck muscles and lubricates your neck joint.

Step-by-Step Instructions

- Sit up tall towards the edge of the chair, lengthen through your spine, and keep your abdominal muscles engaged, shoulders neutral with chest raised.
- Plant your feet flat and firm on the floor at a hip distance apart with toes pointed straight ahead.
- Place your palms face-down on top of your upper thighs and relax your face and limbs
- Take a deep breath in and out through your nose while dropping your chin towards your chest. This is the starting position.
- Maintaining your natural breathing pattern, rotate your head around gently by bringing your left ear towards your left shoulder.
- Keep the rotation going by bringing your head around to the back, gazing up to the ceiling, and keeping the back neck length as long as possible.
- Rotate your head around as gently as possible bringing your right ear towards your right shoulder.
- Roll your head down towards the ground with your chin toward your chest to bring it back to the starting position.
- Repeat steps 4 to 7 five to ten times.
- Repeat the rotations five to time times moving in the opposite direction.
- Bring your head back up gently facing forward after performing your final rotation.

CHAIR CAT-COW STRETCH (CHAIR MARJARYASANA BITILASANA)

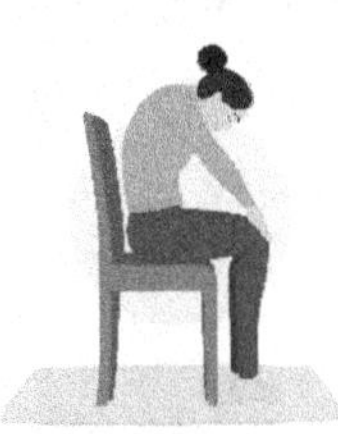

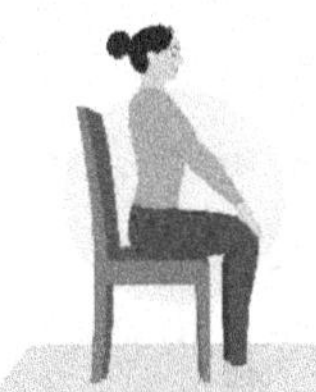

Cat/cow stretch warms up your entire spine, back, shoulders, abdominals, hips, and pelvic floor muscles. It helps an achy back which is very common among older adults. It is good to begin your chair yoga practice with this warm-up because it helps expand your breath, perk up and open your entire body.

Step-by-Step Instructions

- Sit up tall at the edge of the chair, with the spine long, abdominal muscles engaged, shoulders neutral and chest raised.
- Plant your feet flat and firm on the floor at a hip distance apart with toes pointed straight forward.
- Place your palms face-down just above your knees
- When breathing in, bring your chest outward while sticking your hips out behind you.
- Gaze at the ceiling keeping your shoulder blades gently squeezed together.
- Breathe out as you round your chest and spine, scooping your belly inwards, curling under your tailbone as you drop your jawline towards your chest, letting your shoulders approach your ears.
- Repeat for a series of 5-10 cycles.

PELVIC TILTS/CIRCLES

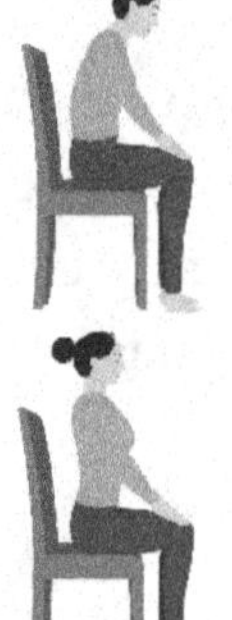

It is always important to warm up your pelvis and lower abs before starting your yoga practice. This is because your pelvic floor region forms the base of your spine and upper body when seated. Tapping into it is a great way to access your organic energy and stay steady all day long. Pelvic circles warm up your spine and lower back, loosen up your lower body and work your pelvic floor and abdominal muscles.

Step-by-Step Instruction

- Sit up tall with your hips towards the edge of the chair, spine long, abdominal muscles engaged, shoulders neutral and chest raised.
- Plant your feet flat and firm on the floor at a hip distance apart with toes pointed straight forward.
- Place your palms face-down on your knees and try to imagine having a marble on your navel and you want it rolled down through your inner thighs.
- Pull your navel inwards imagining you are trying to bring the marble back up in front of your belly towards your navel as you tip your sit bones. Ensure that you isolate just your pelvis. Don't tense your shoulders or arch your upper back.
- Keep rounding and arching your tailbone for about 8 cycles.
- Maintaining the same position, make circles in both clockwise and anticlockwise directions with your pelvis five times for each direction.

FOOT AND ANKLE STRETCH

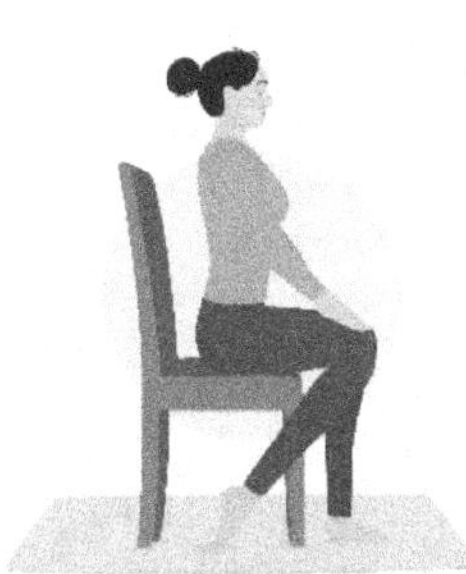

This move helps warm up your ankles, feet, and legs. It also helps lubricate your limb joints increasing their mobility. Foot and ankle stretch makes your feet and ankle muscles more flexible and helps you prevent pain during long walks.

Step-by-Step Instruction

- Begin by sitting up tall in your chair, leaving some space behind you.
- Keep your spine lengthened, shoulders neutral with chest raised, and engage your abdominal muscles.
- Plant your feet flat and firmly on the floor at a hip distance apart with toes pointed straight ahead.
- Place your palms face down on top of your upper thighs and relax your face and limbs
- Extend your left leg straight out in front of you, place your heel on the floor and flex your foot.
- Point your toes towards the ground; ensure that you feel a gentle stretch in the top of your foot
- Keep flexing and pointing your toes towards the floor 5 to 10 times and then bring your left leg back next to the right leg in a gentle manner.
- Repeat steps 4 to 6 with your right leg.
- Do it 5-10 times alternating the legs.

SEATED SHOULDER ROLLS

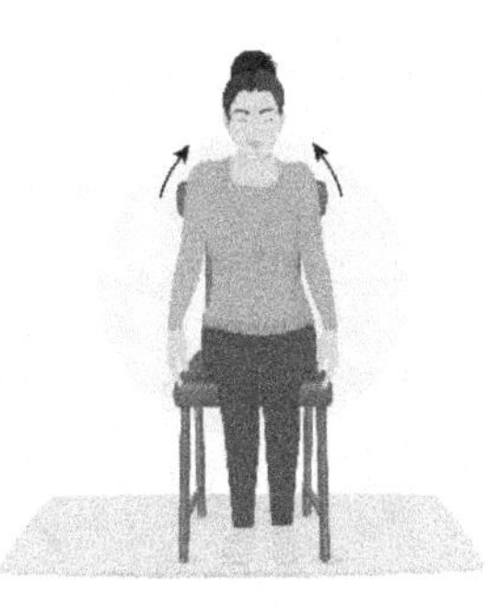

Shoulder rolls help warm up your neck, shoulders, and upper back. They are good for loosening your muscles and lubricating your shoulder joints thus increasing their mobility.

Step-by-Step Instructions

- Sit upright in the chair so that your back isn't leaning on the chair
- Keep your feet flat and firmly planted on the floor at a hip distance apart with your palms on your thighs.
- Take a deep breath in through your nose, lifting both shoulders towards your ears.
- On a breath out, slowly and gently roll both shoulders back and down in a circular motion.
- Continue rolling your shoulders back and down in a smooth and gentle, continuous motion for 5 to 10 rotations.
- Repeat steps 3 and 4 in the alternate direction for 5-10 rotations

SEATED SIDE BEND POSE

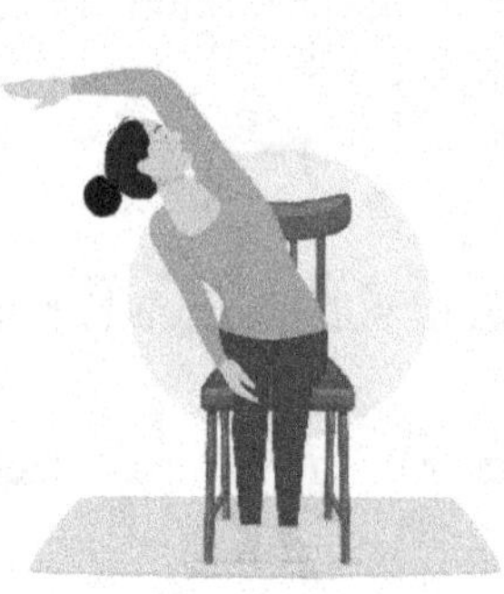

This pose stretches the neck, shoulders, back, arms and obliques. It is a good warm-up exercise for gaining joint mobility and flexibility in your arms, shoulders, and upper body muscles.

Step-by-Step Instruction

- Sit up tall in the chair so that your back isn't leaning on it
- Keep your feet flat and firmly planted on the floor at a hip distance apart with your palms on your thighs.
- Remaining firmly seated on the chair with both your shin bones planted on it, place your right palm face-down on your left thigh and reach your left hand up and over to the left facing forward and tilting your torso over slightly to the right.

- Hold the pose for a few seconds (for one deep and complete breath). You should feel the stretch on the left side of the torso.
- Release yourself slowly back to a neutral position with your spine upright and arms down by your sides.
- Switch to the opposite side and repeat.

SUN SALUTATIONS

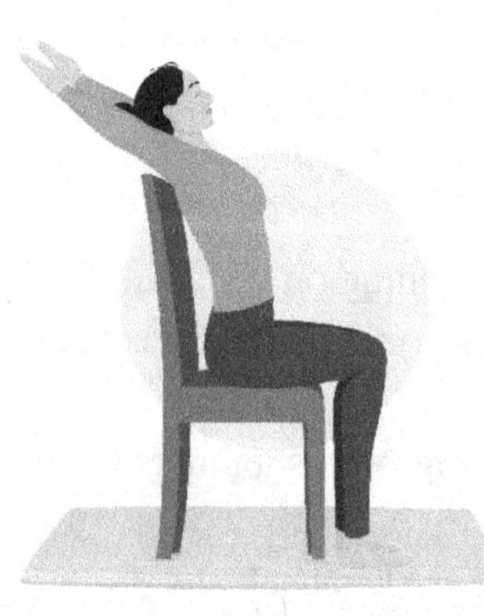

Performing sun salutations enhances better blood circulation, breath expansion, and increased flexibility. They bring warmth and heat into our bodies releasing the tension in our shoulders, head, and neck. The following sun salutation sequence is a great way to warm up.

Step-by-Step Instructions

- Sit up in the chair leaving some space behind you
- Keep your feet flat and firmly planted on the floor with your knees slightly wider than hip-width apart and palms face-down on top of your thighs.
- On a breath in, sweep your hands outwards to your sides and then lift them overhead.
- On a breath out, slowly and gently lower your hand back to the thighs leaning forward while flattening your back.
- Fold over as you breathe in and out until your hands rest on your shins or floor.

- Breathe in and come back to the starting position with a flat back and hands resting on your thighs then breathe out.
- Repeat steps 3 to 5 for 5 -10 times.

MARCHING FLOW

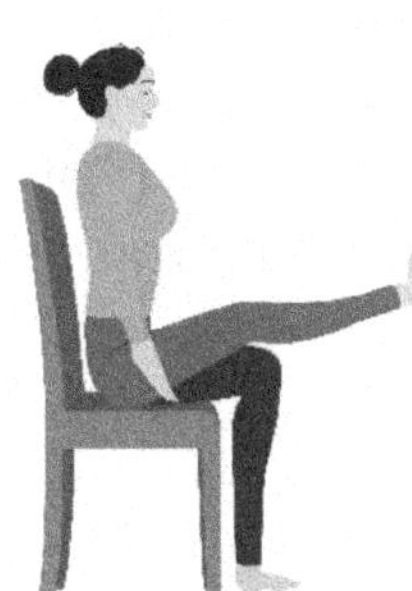

Most seniors spent most of their time seated. Staying seated for a prolonged period makes you feel restricted and tied up in your hips and lower back. The matching flow gets your legs moving, boosting metabolism and working them out. Most yoga exercises concentrate more on large muscle groups and this pose also gets our lower half warmed up. It works on your core, external rotators, quadriceps, and inner thighs.

Step-by-Step Instruction

- Sit tall in the chair, with your back straight leaving some space behind you so that your back isn't leaning on it.
- Keep your feet flat and firmly planted on the floor at a hip distance apart with your palms on your thighs.
- Breathe in as you straighten your right leg out in front of you; ensure to engage your quadriceps and lengthen behind your knee.
- Breathe out and bend your knee to open your right hip as you rest the right outer ankle on your left knee (you may be required to use your hand to help place the foot on your knee and open the leg).
- Breathe in and slowly and gently extend the leg back forward, then breathe out and gently lower the foot and put it on the floor.
- Repeat the sequence alternating the legs.

<h1>KNEE SWINGS</h1>

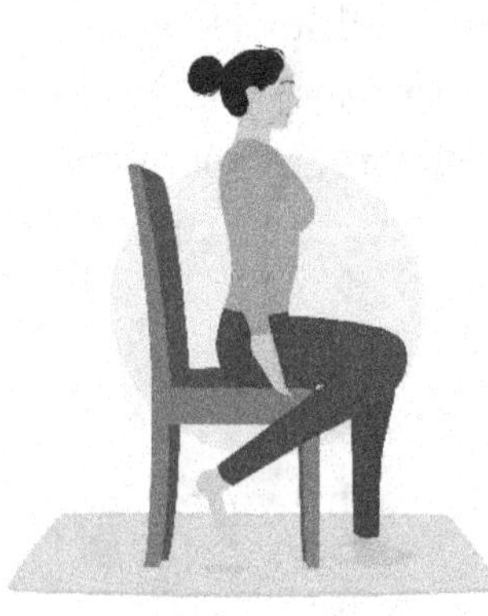

This is among the few poses that are done quickly. If you can't reach under your knee with your back straight, then just sit back in the chair and do the kicks swinging back and forth at a speed you are comfortable with. This warm-up exercise helps lubricate the knee joint thus increasing mobility and range of motion in the knees.

Step-by-Step Instructions
- Sit up tall in the chair leaving some space behind you.
- Keep your back straight, shoulders neutral, and engage your abdominal muscles
- Plant your feet flat and firmly on the floor at a hip distance apart with toes pointed straight ahead and arms hanging by your sides.
- Clasp both hands under your right knee while maintaining a straight back.
- While holding your knee, begin kicking your leg out back and forth
- Repeat alternating the legs.

OUR EXCLUSIVE
ADVANCED PROGRAM

INTENSE SIDE STRETCH (PARSVOTTANASANA)

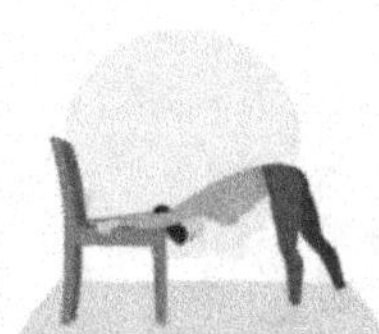

This pose engages the muscles of your shoulders, back, arms, hips, and legs. It is helpful in stretching and strengthening your legs and gaining flexibility in the hip muscles and mobility of your hip joint. Although this stretch may be intense at the beginning, it is very functional and can help you move more freely in daily life.

Step-by-Step Instructions
- Stand up tall in front of the chair facing it. Your feet should be parallel to each other at hip-width apart.
- Take a deep breath in and out then hold the chair seat with both hands. Ensure that you feel stable and relaxed.
- Make one step backward with your right foot and place it down at about a leg's length behind you or away from your left foot.
- Keep your back nice, relaxed, and lengthened, and both legs straight engaging the quadriceps and the area above the kneecaps.
- Keeping your back straight, slowly tilt your torso forward as if you are laying your chest over your front thigh until it is parallel to the ground.
- Hold this position for about 5-10 deep inhales and exhales
- Repeat for the opposite leg.

CHAIR BOAT POSE (CHAIR NAVASANA)

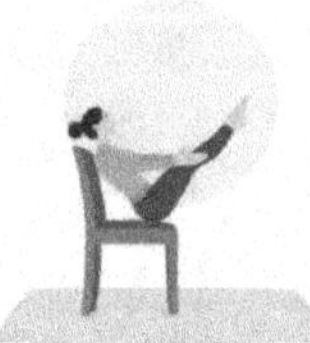

Chair Navasana works out the abdominals, hamstrings, hips, and quadriceps. Try it out if you want to strengthen these muscles.

Step-by-Step Instructions
- Sit up tall and comfortable towards the edge of the chair with your spine erect and relaxed, feet flat on the floor at about hip-width apart.
- Rest your hands on your upper thighs just above your knees and take a deep breath in through your nose and slowly exhale.
- Lean back engaging your abdominals and lift your legs off the ground with your feet flexed.
- Hold this position for about 3-5 deep breaths
- Gently release the legs back to the ground one at a time.
- Repeat.

CHAIR GODDESS TWIST (CHAIR PARIVRTTA UTKATA KONASANA)

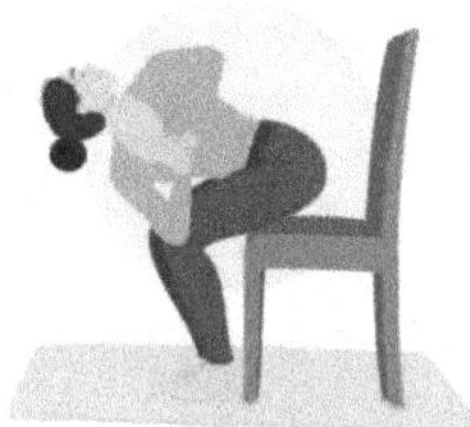

This pose engages and works out the sides of your torso, your inner thighs, arms, and hips. It is good for stretching and strengthening the oblique muscles and arms. It also helps boost your mood and confidence.

Step-by-Step Instructions
- Sit up tall and comfortable towards the edge of the chair with your spine erect and relaxed, feet planted firmly on the floor at about hip-width apart.
- Rest your hands on your upper thighs just above your knees and take a deep breath in through your nose and slowly exhale.
- Widen your legs such that each leg gets to either side of the chair.
- Slowly and gently twist your upper body towards the left, lifting your right arm up above your head and lowering your left arm down towards your left ankle with your palms facing forward.
- Look up towards your right hand and gaze at the palm
- Hold there for 5-10 deep breaths
- Gently bring your legs back and your right arms down to release the pose
- Repeat.

WARRIOR III (VIRABHADRASANA III)

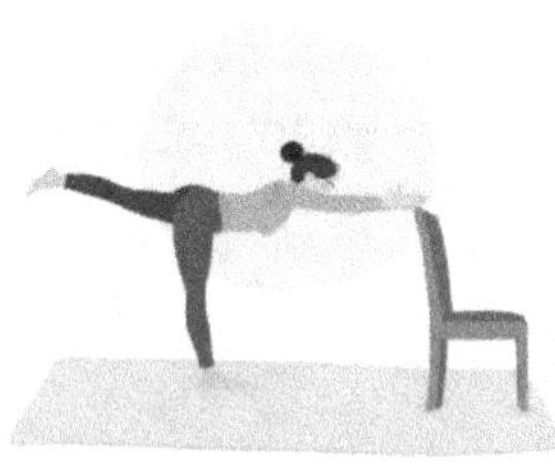

Chair warrior III is more challenging but super fun to perform. It requires you to have a lot of abdominal control and strength in the buttocks. You can perform this exercise when you are in need of some focus and energy or want to challenge your balance and improve it. This pose helps work out your buttocks, core, and back.

Step-by-Step Instructions
- Begin by sitting up tall towards the edge of the chair with your butt in the middle of the seat, so that you can easily pivot to the left and sit on your right side.
- Take a deep breath in through your nose and exhale slowly.
- Gently inch over towards the left side of the chair with your right hamstring flat on the seat of the chair, right knee bent and straighten out your left leg and extend it back behind you and ensure that your toes are pressed firmly on the floor.

- Bent forward until you can raise your back leg off the floor.
- Stretch your arms straight out to the sides with palms facing down. You can stretch your arms straight back too.
- Hold there for about 5-10 deep inhales and exhales.
- Repeat on the opposite side.

CROSS-LEGGED TWIST

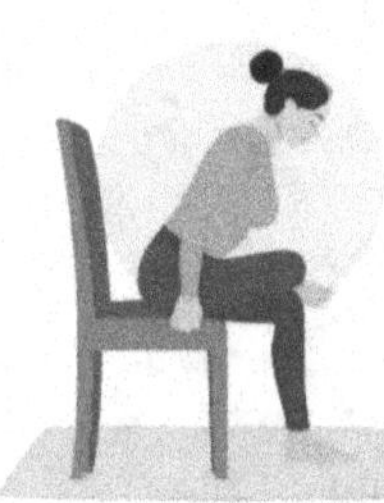

This pose engages the back, legs, and hips. It is helpful in gaining muscle flexibility and joint mobility in the spine and hips. It also helps relieve tension and stiffness. Thanks to its twisting motion.

Step-by-Step Instructions

- Sit up tall in the chair leaving some space behind you. Plant your feet flat and firmly on the floor at a hip distance apart with your palms facing down on the upper side of your thighs.
- Take a deep breath in and out then bring your entire right leg and cross it on top of your left thigh.
- Let your left-hand rest on your right thigh as the right-hand rest on the chair seat behind you
- Breathe in as you lengthen your spine, then breathe out and twist your upper body towards the right. Look behind and go as far as you can.
- Hold there for 3-5 deep breaths.
- Unwind from the twist slowly and gently, returning to the center and uncrossing your leg, putting it back on the floor.
- Repeat for the opposite side.

ADVANCED HAMSTRING STRETCH

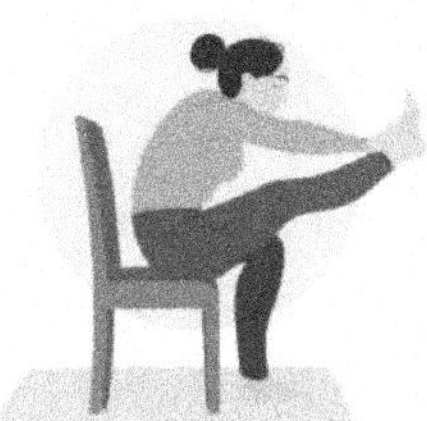

This stretch is quite intense but good for you. Not only does it open up your entire back but it also engages your core and lower back. Advanced hamstring stretch works out your hamstrings, abs, arms, and legs. It is the best exercise for stretching your hamstrings, inner thighs, and legs.

Step-by-Step Instructions
- Sit up tall and comfortable towards the edge of the chair with your spine erect and relaxed, feet flat on the floor at about hip-width apart.
- Rest your hands on your upper thighs just above your knees and take a deep breath in through your nose and slowly exhale.
- Hold your right ankle and straighten your leg out in front of you. Hold the pose for about 3-5 deep breaths.
- Now, try lifting the leg up towards your face, while maintaining a straight back. Hold for another 3-5 deep breaths.
- Sit upright again and try to open the leg to the right side for another 3-5 deep breaths
- For a hamstring and IT band stretch, bring the leg across the midsection and then to the left. Hold this position for another 3-5 deep breaths then release the leg.
- Repeat for the opposite leg.

HIGH LUNGE

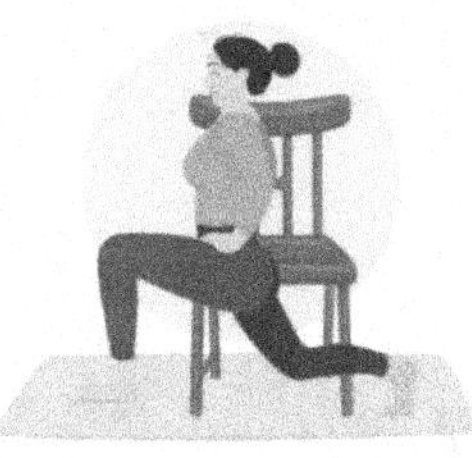

This pose works out your quads, hips, hamstrings, and glutes. It is good for deep full-body stretching and strengthening. It improves blood circulation and boosts metabolism.

Step-by-Step Instructions
- Stand up tall sideways behind a chair. Your feet should be parallel to each other at hip-width apart.
- Take a deep breath in and out then hold on to the chair back with your right hand and make a leg's length step backward with your left leg.
- Lunge the right knee deeply until the thigh becomes almost parallel to the chair seat.
- Ensure to keep the knee above the ankle to protect it.
- Press through your left knee firmly and extend your left knee behind. Keep your right glute muscles and abdominals deeply engaged and anchor the whole right foot to the ground. Lift your left hand up towards the ceiling.

- Hold there for about 5-10 deep breaths
- Return to an upright standing position and repeat for the opposite leg.

TREE

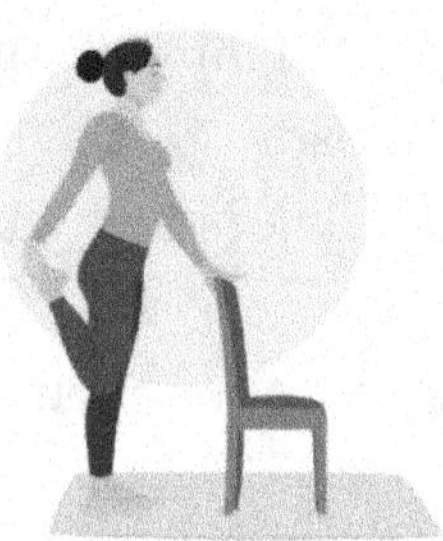

Tree pose works your hips and legs. It helps stretch and strengthen the muscles of the standing leg and improve mobility and flexibility of the hip joint. This exercise also helps improve body awareness and balance.

Step-by-Step Instructions
- Stand up tall sideways behind a chair. Your feet should be parallel to each other at hip-width apart.
- Take a deep breath in and out then hold on to the chair back with your left hand.
- Place your right hand on your hip and bend your right knee.
- Let your right heel rest on your left leg while the toes of your right foot touch the floor.
- Try to move your right foot up such that its sole rests on your left leg just below the knee
- Once you feel stable, put your hands together in front of your chest. You can also try to lift them up or put them together above your head.
- Hold here for a few relaxed breaths
- Repeat with your opposite leg.

RAISED KNEE BALANCE

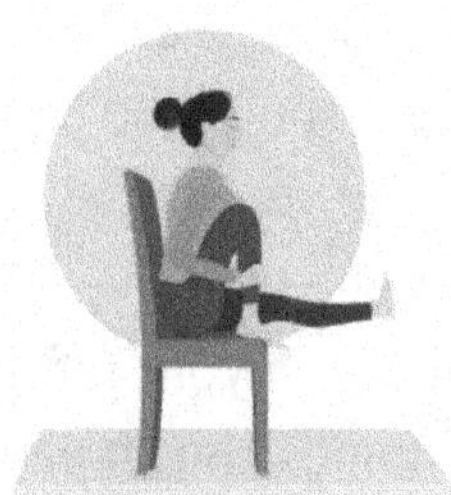

This posture works your hips, knee joints, and legs. It helps improve flexibility and mobility of the hip and knee joints. It also strengthens your leg muscles thus improving your stability and balance.

Step-by-Step Instruction
- Stand up tall in front of the chair with its side facing you. Your feet should be parallel to each other at hip-width apart.
- Take a deep breath in and out then hold the back of the chair with one hand for support. Ensure that you feel stable and relaxed.
- Slowly and mindfully lift the leg that is closest to the chair and put its foot on top of the chair seat. Ensure that your whole foot is on the seat.
- Hold here for a few relaxed breaths. You may try lifting your hand an inch off the chair if you feel your balance is good.

- You may also use a block for placing the foot if the chair is too high and just use the chair for support to hold onto.
- Slowly and gently return the leg to the floor and do the same with the other leg.
- Repeat, alternating the legs.

TIPPY TOES

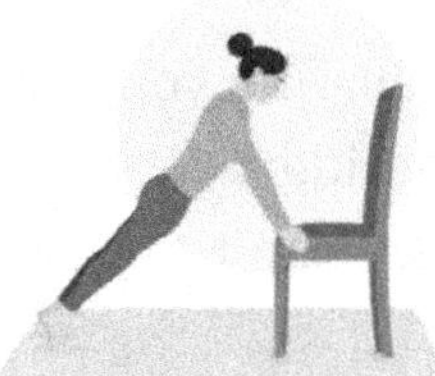

This pose will work out your feet, ankle, and calves. It helps strengthen your calf muscles, improve ankle joints and feet flexibility and mobility and improve balance and stability.

Step-by-Step Instruction

- Stand up tall behind a chair facing its back about a foot away from it. Your feet should be parallel to each other at hip-width apart.
- Take a deep breath in and out then hold the back of the chair with both hands. Ensure that you feel stable and relaxed.
- Rise onto the tips of your toes.
- Slowly lower your heels to the ground. Ensure that you don't feel any impact when your heels touch the floor.
- Raise your heels again and lower them in the same way.
- Repeat raising and lowering your heels as slowly and as quietly as possible

COOLING DOWN

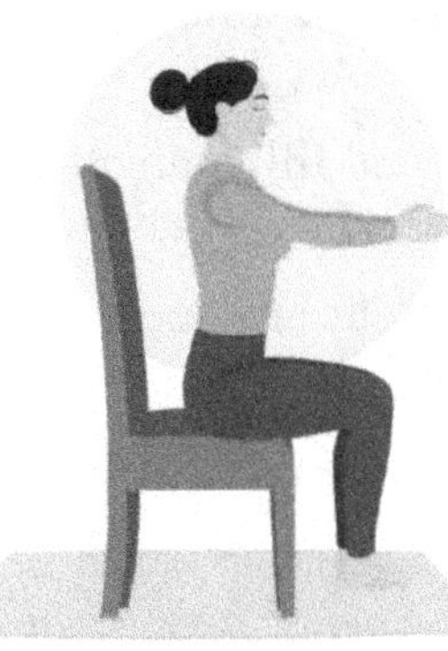

- Sit tall and comfortable in your chair
- Bring your palms together and rub them against each other until you feel warmth in them
- Cup them slightly and gently place them over your face covering your eyes. You may close your eyes or keep them open.
- Feel the warmth of the palms on your eyes. Ensure not to put pressure on your eyeballs.
- Hold the pose for about three to five minutes.

COOLING BREATH (SITKARI)

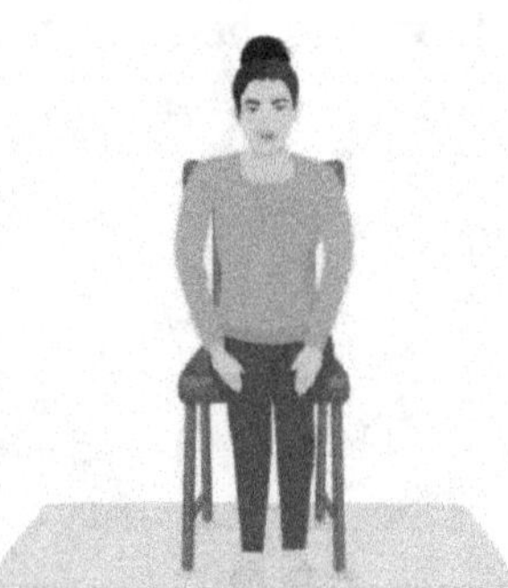

- Sit up tall in the chair with your hips towards the edge of the chair, back straight, your feet planted firmly on the floor at a hip-width apart.
- Take a few natural breaths in and out to center yourself.
- With your lips open, close your teeth by bringing your lower and upper teeth together and inhale through them producing a soft hissing sound.
- Release the teeth and close your mouth as you breathe out through the nose
- Repeat until you feel a nice cooling effect that eases your body and mind.

FINAL RELAXATION AND MEDITATION

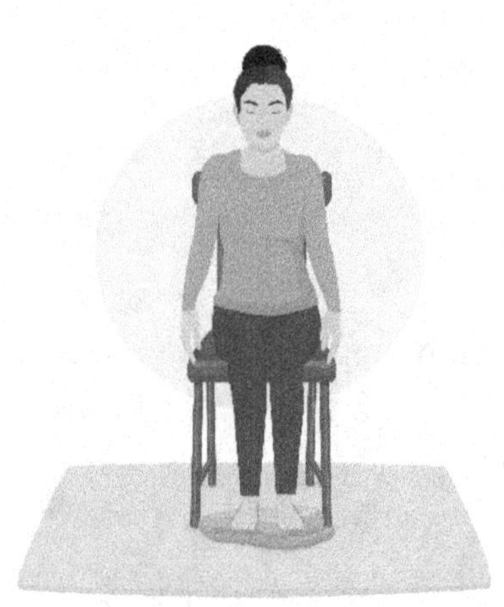

- Sit up tall and comfortable at the edge of the chair with your spine erect and relaxed, feet flat on the floor at about hip-width apart. Raise your feet using a bolster or a folded blanket if they can't touch the ground when seated.
- Rest your hands on your upper thighs just above your knees and relax your entire body.
- Close your eyes and imagine a vibrant beautiful rainbow in the sky. It is so close that you can see all of its colors perfectly.
- Take a deep breath and as you inhale, visualize the color red. Keep your body relaxed and let go of any tension as you exhale.
- Take a deep breath and as you inhale, visualize the color orange. Breathe out and let go of any negative emotions.
- Take a deep breath and as you inhale, visualize the color yellow. Breathe out and relax your mind.
- Take a deep breath and as you inhale, visualize the color green. Breathe out and find a state of tranquility within yourself.
- Take a deep breath and as you inhale, visualize the color blue. Breathe out and fill yourself with love.
- Take a deep breath and as you inhale, visualize the color Indigo. Breathe out and locate your most hidden inner self.
- Take a deep breath and as you inhale, visualize the color violet. Breathe out and stay with your most intimate self.
- You are now on your deepest mental level.
- Now focus on any goal that you want to achieve in your workout or life. Be inspired by yourself.
- Prepare to come out from meditation. As you come out, you will feel a sense of peace and cleansing and your body will be in perfect harmony and ready to act.

RECIPES

DAY 1

BREAKFAST: **Bacon & Eggs**

Prep Time: 7 mins
Cook Time: 13 mins

Ingredients: 2 large eggs (or 4 small), 1 slice of deli turkey bacon, 1 tomato, tablespoon chopped fresh chives, salt and ground black pepper to taste

Preparation:

-Mix the eggs, turkey, and bacon in a bowl and season with salt and pepper. Spoon into a small baking dish. Add some oil on top of the egg mixture. Bake at 400°F for about 12 minutes or until firm and slightly toasted around the edges
-Top with some chopped tomato, chives and salt and pepper. Enjoy!

LUNCH: **Beef & Cheddar Biscuits with Salsa**

Prep Time: 10 mins
Cook Time: 30 mins

Ingredients: 3/4 cup whole wheat flour (or all-purpose flour), 1 tablespoon baking powder, 1/2 teaspoon sea salt. 2 tablespoons butter, cut into small pieces., 1 cup grated cheddar cheese (or to taste), 1 cup ranch dressing (or to taste), a pinch of cayenne pepper (or to taste), 1/2 teaspoon chilli powder, 1/2 cup chopped fresh cilantro (or to taste), a pinch of ground black pepper, 1 beef steak, thawed (8 - 12 ounces)

Preparation:

-Preheat the oven to 400° F. Grease a baking sheet and set aside
-In a bowl, mix flour, salt and baking powder. Add in the butter, cheese, ranch dressing, chilli powder, cayenne pepper and cilantro, and then mix with a fork. Form into a 1/2-inch-thick patty and place on the prepared baking sheet
-Place in the preheated oven for about 20 minutes or until browned. Slice into 1/2-inch-thick slices, then. serve while warm
-Enjoy!

DINNER: **Grilled Beef & Asparagus**

Prep Time: 15 mins
Cook Time: 25 mins

Ingredients: 2 pounds asparagus, 3 pounds grass-fed beef tenderloin, thinly sliced (can use ground beef for a similar flavor), 1 tablespoon sea salt, 1 tablespoon ground black pepper, 1 cup panko bread crumbs (or to taste), 2 tablespoons olive oil, 1 tablespoon paprika, a pinch of cayenne pepper (or to taste), a pinch of turmeric (optional)

Preparation:
-Preheat the oven to 400° F. Line a baking sheet with foil and set aside
-Toss the asparagus in a bowl with the sea salt and ground black pepper, then set aside
-Arrange the beef slices on top of each other on a large baking dish. Season with salt, pepper and cayenne (or to taste). Top with some olive oil and paprika. Bake at 400° F for about 30 minutes or until the beef is slightly browned.
-While the beef is cooking, chop up asparagus into bite-size pieces and place in a small skillet over medium heat. Add in some oil. Toss to coat the asparagus. Stir in the turmeric (optional)
-Arrange the roasted beef over top of each serving plate. Spoon some warm asparagus on top of the beef, and season with a pinch of sea salt and ground black pepper to taste then. serve while warm
-Enjoy!

DAY 2

BREAKFAST: **American Pancakes**

Prep Time: 15 mins
Cook Time: 12 mins

Ingredients: American Pancakes, all-purpose flour, baking powder, salt, sugar, egg, milk, butter

Preparation:
-In a large bowl, whisk together the flour, baking powder, salt and sugar
-In a separate bowl, whisk together the egg and milk
-Stir the wet ingredients into the dry ingredients until just combined
-Melt the butter in a large skillet over medium heat
-For each pancake, spoon about two tablespoons of batter onto the skillet
-Cook for one to two minutes or until bubbles form and pop and the edges are dry
-Flip and cook for an additional one to two minutes
-Serve with butter and syrup

LUNCH: **American Fried Rice**

Prep Time: 15 mins
Cook Time: 12 mins

Ingredients: American Fried Rice, rice, eggs, green onions, soy sauce, vegetable oil, frozen peas and carrots

Preparation:
-Cook the rice according to the package directions
-In a separate skillet, scramble the eggs
-Stir in the green onions, soy sauce and vegetable oil
-Cook for about one minute or until the eggs are just set
-Stir in the cooked rice and frozen peas, and carrots
-Cook for about five minutes or until heated through
Serves: American recipes

DINNER: **American Shepherd's Pie**

Prep Time: 15 mins
Cook Time: 40 mins

Ingredients: American Shepherd's Pie, potatoes, milk, butter, salt and pepper, ground beef, onion, garlic powder, can (15 oz) corn, drained

Preparation:
-Peel and chop the potatoes
-Place them in a large pot and cover with water
-Bring to a boil and cook for about 15 minutes or until tender
-Drain the potatoes and return them to the pot
-Add the milk, butter, salt and pepper
-Mash the potatoes until they are smooth
-In a separate skillet over medium heat, cook the ground beef until browned
-Stir in the onion and garlic powder
-Stir in the corn and cook for an additional five minutes
-Preheat the oven to 350 degrees Fahrenheit
-Spread the mashed potatoes over the ground beef mixture in the skillet
-Bake for about 20 minutes or until the potatoes are golden brown

DAY 3

BREAKFAST: American Banana Bread

Prep Time: 15 mins
Cook Time: 40 mins

Ingredients: American Banana Bread, flour, sugar, baking soda, salt, canola oil, mashed bananas (2-3), vanilla extract

Preparation:
-Heat the oven to 350 degrees Fahrenheit and grease a loaf pan
-In a large bowl, mix the flour, sugar and baking soda
-Stir in the canola oil and mashed bananas until just combined
-Beat in the vanilla extract until smooth
-Pour into the loaf pan and bake for about 30. minutes or until golden brown and a toothpick inserted in the middle comes out clean

LUNCH: American Meatloaf

Prep Time: 20 mins
Cook Time: 50 mins

Ingredients: American Meatloaf, onions, garlic powder, beef, beef bouillon cubes, can (15 oz) tomato sauce, salt and pepper

Preparation:
-In a large skillet over medium heat, brown the onions and garlic powder in a little oil until the onions are soft and aromatic
-Add the ground beef and brown it on all sides, then add the tomato sauce and bouillon cubes
-Season with salt and pepper to taste then. reduce the heat and simmer for about five minutes or until thickened
-Preheat the oven to 350 degrees Fahrenheit
-Grease a loaf pan and spoon the meat mixture into it
-Bake for about 20 minutes or until heated through and a toothpick inserted in the middle comes out clean

DINNER: American Lasagna

Prep Time: 15 mins

Cook Time: 25 mins

Ingredients: Lasagna noodles, ground beef, garlic powder, onion powder, Italian. seasoning, salt and pepper, broth, cottage cheese, ricotta cheese

Preparation:

-In a large skillet over medium heat, brown the ground beef with the garlic powder, onion powder and Italian seasoning
-Season with salt and pepper to taste
-Stir in the broth and simmer for an additional five minutes or until thickened
-In a small saucepan over medium heat, cook the lasagna noodles according to the package directions
-Stir the cottage cheese and ricotta cheese into the ground beef mixture. pour the mixture over the noodles
-Spread the lasagna in a 9 x 13 pan and cook for about 25 minutes or until bubbly and a toothpick inserted in the middle comes out clean

DAY 4

BREAKFAST: **American Sausage Gravy**

Prep Time: 15 mins
Cook Time: 15 mins

Ingredients: Flour, butter, cooked sausage, salt and pepper, milk

Preparation:

-In a large saucepan over medium heat, melt the butter and sprinkle in the flour
-Whisk until smooth then. cook for about one minute
-Stir in the milk and boil until thickened
-Stir in the cooked sausage and cook an additional five minutes
-Season to taste with salt and pepper

LUNCH: **American Chicken Cheese Casserole**

Prep Time: 15 mins
Cook Time: 25 mins

Ingredients: chicken breasts, low-sodium chicken broth, garlic powder, onion powder, Italian seasoning, salt and pepper, and egg whites (2). cheese, bread crumbs

Preparation:
-Preheat the oven to 350 degrees Fahrenheit and lightly grease a large casserole dish
-Cook the chicken breasts in a skillet over medium heat for about five minutes on each side or until cooked through, then cut into small cubes
-Heat the broth over medium heat in a large saucepan with the garlic powder, onion powder, and Italian seasoning, then season with salt and pepper to taste
-Stir in the chicken, egg whites and cheese until combined. pour into the casserole dish and sprinkle with bread crumbs
-Bake for about 15 minutes or until golden brown and a toothpick inserted in the middle comes out clean
Serves: American recipes

DINNER: **American Spicy Black Bean Soup**

Prep Time: 10 mins
Cook Time: 20 mins

Ingredients: black beans, salsa, corn, jalapeno pepper, garlic powder, chili powder, salt and pepper, and vegetable oil.

Preparation:
-Heat the pan on medium heat and cook the salsa, jalapeno and corn in a little oil until the corn is just tender
-Stir in the black beans, garlic powder, chili powder and salt and pepper to taste
-In a small saucepan, add the vegetable oil and bring to a slight boil, then turn off the heat
-Pour into a blender with half of the soup mixture into it, then blend until smooth
-Pour into two bowls, pour an equal amount of hot sauce and garnish with an equal amount of sour cream.

DAY 5

BREAKFAST: **American French Toast Casserole**

Prep Time: 15 mins
Cook Time: 45 mins

Ingredients: French bread, eggs (6), milk, cinnamon sugar, topping (1/4 cup brown sugar, 1/4 cup of melted butter), vanilla extract.

Preparation:

-Slice the French bread into thick slices then. place in a 9 x 13 pan
-Whisk together the eggs, milk, cinnamon and vanilla extract then. pour over the French bread
-Spread evenly and let soak for about 20 minutes or until the liquid has been absorbed by the bread
-Bake for about 20 minutes or until puffy
-While baking, prepare the topping by mixing the brown sugar and melted butter in a small bowl, then drizzle over the casserole
-After the casserole has finished baking, spread the topping over it then. bake for an additional 10 minutes or until golden brown and a toothpick inserted in the middle comes out clean

LUNCH: **American Creamy Chicken**

Prep Time: 10 mins
Cook Time: 20 mins

Ingredients: chicken breasts, green beans, salt and pepper, garlic powder, can (10 oz) cream of mushroom soup, sour cream.

Preparation:

-Heat the saucepan on medium heat and cook the green beans for about three minutes and then season with salt and pepper
-Add in the chicken breasts, then season with garlic powder, add in the cream of mushroom soup and simmer for an additional five minutes or until cooked through. Season to taste

-In a small saucepan over medium heat, cook the remaining ingredients until heated. Serve with the chicken breasts

DINNER: **American Barbecue Meatballs**

Prep Time: 15 mins
Cook Time: 25 mins

Ingredients: ground beef, eggs (2), barbecue sauce (1 bottle), garlic powder, onion powder, salt and pepper, and bread crumbs.

Preparation:
-Mix the ground beef and egg in a bowl until combined. season with garlic powder, onion powder, salt and pepper
-In a large saucepan, heat the sauce to a boil, then turn off the heat
-In the same saucepan over medium heat, cook the bread crumbs and barbecue sauce until heated. Pour into a bowl and set aside
-In a large saucepan over medium heat, cook the meatballs in the barbecue sauce until cooked through
-Place an equal amount of meatballs on each bun and cover with an equal amount of barbecue sauce and top with the bread crumbs
-Serve warm

DAY 6

BREAKFAST: **Apple Oatmeal**

Prep Time: 10 mins
Cook Time: 15 mins

Ingredients: apple juice concentrate (1 oz), cinnamon, rolled oats, raisins (dried), nuts/seeds, brown sugar, butter, water, and One whole apple.

Preparation:
-Heat a saucepan on medium heat. Add in the apple juice concentrate, cinnamon, rolled oats, raisins and nuts/seeds
-Add the butter to a saucepan and. melt until just starting to brown, then pour over the top of the oatmeal mixture
-In a separate small saucepan, add some water and bring to a boil, then set aside

-Cut the apple in half, then slice it into thin pieces. Melt together the sugar and butter in a small saucepan over medium heat, then pour evenly over the top of each serving bowl of oatmeal. Add the sliced apple to each serving dish and. serve immediately

LUNCH: **American Chicken Sandwich**

Prep Time: 10 mins
Cook Time: 10 mins

Ingredients: chicken breast, salt and pepper, vegetable oil, American deli cheese (Cabot 50% cheese), bread, sandwich rolls (2), mayonnaise, chili powder or hot sauce, lettuce (1 head), sliced tomato.

Preparation:
-Slice the chicken breasts in half then. pound flat and season with salt and pepper on both sides
-Heat a frying pan over medium heat and cook the chicken for about four minutes on each side, then set aside on a plate
-Spread an equal amount of mayonnaise over the inside of each bun, then layer an equal amount of cheese over each bun
-Place the meat in two buns, then top with an equal amount of lettuce, sliced tomato, chilli powder or hot sauce and roll up

DINNER: **American Fried Chicken**

Prep Time: 10 mins
Cook Time: 15 mins

Ingredients: chicken breasts, vegetable oil, flour (1 cup), eggs (6), milk, salt and pepper, corn starch mixed with water, flour (1/3 cup), bread crumbs, and spices of your choice.

Preparation:
-Cut the chicken breasts into small pieces then. season with salt and pepper
-In a large saucepan, heat the oil over medium heat -Whisk together the flour, eggs, milk, salt, and pepper in a bowl. Pour into a shallow dish -In another shallow dish, add the corn starch mixed with water. Pour into a third shallow dish the bread crumbs mixed with spices of your choice
-Dip each piece of chicken into the flour mixture, then the corn starch mixture and the bread crumb mixture -Place the chicken pieces into the hot oil and fry for about two minutes on each side or until golden brown
-Remove from the oil and drain on paper towels

DAY 7

BREAKFAST: **Blueberry Toast**

Prep Time: 20 mins
Cook Time: 5 mins

Ingredients: blueberry jam (1 tablespoon), whole wheat bread (2 slices), butter, eggs, milk or cream.

Preparation:

-In a small saucepan over medium heat, bring the blueberry jam to a boil, then turn off the heat and set aside
-Combine the egg(s) or milk and one slice of bread in a small bowl, then whisk to combine. Then dip the other piece of bread into the mixture and fry in a little butter until golden brown on both sides. Serve with the blueberry jam

LUNCH: **American Tacos**

Prep Time: 30 mins
Cook Time: 15 mins

Ingredients: ground beef, onions, bell pepper, cheddar cheese (4 oz), salsa (1 can), sour cream, tortillas (2), 2-3 tablespoons of cheese.

Preparation:

-Heat a frying pan over medium-high heat and cook the ground beef until cooked through, then drain on a paper towel and set aside
-While the meat is cooking, sauté the onion and bell pepper in a saucepan over medium heat for about 5 minutes, then add the salsa and allow to simmer for an additional eight minutes or until the vegetables have softened enough to break apart easily, then stir together with the ground beef
-Heat a frying pan over medium heat and add a bit of oil, then evenly spread the meat mixture in the pan
-When the tortillas are baked and hot, add two or three tablespoons of cheese to each tortilla, then fold into a taco shape and roll up in each tortilla. Serve warm with spoonful of sour cream on top

DINNER: **American Chili**

Prep Time: 20 mins
Cook Time: 30 mins

Ingredients: ground beef, onions, garlic, kidney beans (1 can), diced tomatoes (1 can), chilli powder, salt and pepper, and cumin.

Preparation:

-In a large saucepan over medium-high heat, cook the ground beef until browned, then add the onions and garlic and sauté for an additional five minutes
-Stir in the kidney beans, diced tomatoes, chilli powder, salt and pepper and cumin then. bring to a boil
-Reduce the heat to low and simmer for about 30 minutes or until the flavours have melded together
-Serve with a dollop of sour cream on top, and enjoy!

DAY 8

BREAKFAST: American Breakfast Casserole

Prep Time: 10 mins Longer Time Start: 20 mins

Ingredients: bacon (4 strips), cream of mushroom soup, butter, eggs (2), onions (2), American cheese slice, salsa, pepper jack cheese slice, salt.

Preparation:

-Heat a frying pan over medium heat and cook the bacon until crisp. Drain on a paper towel and set aside on a plate or in the frying pan. Set aside the bacon fat to saute the other ingredients.
-Whisk together the cream of mushroom soup, eggs and butter then. add the onions and sauté in the bacon fat for about 3 minutes or until they start to become translucent
-Pour the egg mixture into a baking dish big enough to fit all of the ingredients, then crumble the bacon on top and stir in
-Top with American cheese slices, salsa, and pepper jack cheese.
-Bake at 350 degrees Fahrenheit for about 20 minutes or until the eggs are firm, and the cheese is melted and bubbly.

LUNCH: **American Club Sandwich**

Prep Time: 15 mins

Ingredients: turkey or chicken breast, bacon (3 strips), mayo, avocado, tomato, lettuce, whole wheat bread.

Preparation:
-Cook the bacon in a frying pan over medium heat until crisp, then drain on a paper towel and set aside
-Slice the turkey or chicken breast into thin strips then. add to the frying pan and cook until browned
-Spread mayo on two slices of whole wheat bread then. top with avocado, tomato, lettuce and chicken or turkey strips
-Top with the other slice of bread and cut into four equal pieces

DINNER: **American Shepherd's Pie**

Prep Time: 30 mins
Cook Time: 45 mins

Ingredients: ground beef, onion, garlic, carrots, corn (1 can), green beans (1 can), tomato paste, beef broth, red wine, thyme, and potatoes.

Preparation:
-In a large saucepan over medium-high heat, cook the ground beef until browned, then add the onion and garlic and sauté for an additional five minutes
-Stir in the carrots, corn, green beans, tomato paste, beef broth, red wine and thyme then. bring to a boil
-Reduce the heat to low and simmer for about 30 minutes or until the vegetables are tender
-Meanwhile, peel and chop the potatoes then. add them to a pot of boiling water and cook for about 10 minutes or until they are soft
-Drain the potatoes then. add them to a large bowl and mash with some butter, milk and salt and pepper to taste
-Preheat the oven to 350 degrees Fahrenheit then. spread the mashed potatoes over the top of the beef and vegetable mixture in the saucepan
-Bake in the oven for about 15 minutes or until the potatoes are browned and bubbly

DAY 9

BREAKFAST: **American Frittata**

Prep Time: 10 mins
Cook Time: 20 mins

Ingredients: Asparagus (1 bunch), Swiss cheese (1 bunch), mushrooms, olive oil, onions, salt and pepper, and eggs.

Preparation:
-Heat a large frying pan over medium heat then. cook the asparagus in it for about ten minutes or until soft
-While the asparagus is cooking, cook the mushrooms in a saucepan over medium heat for about 8 minutes, then add in the olive oil and onions and sauté for an additional five minutes
-In a large bowl, pour beaten eggs. Add the Swiss cheese, salt and pepper, then mix well
-Add the cooked mushrooms and asparagus to the large bowl and pour in some olive oil until each egg portion has been coated. Pour into greased baking dish.
-In a separate medium-sized frying pan, sauté the onions and mushrooms for about five minutes, and top with salt and pepper. Add the Swiss cheese and continue to saute until melted
-Bake in a 350 degrees Fahrenheit oven for about 20 minutes
-Bing out of the oven, serve and enjoy.

LUNCH: **Chicken Salad**

Prep Time: 10 mins

Ingredients: Chicken breast, bacon (2 strips), green onion, lettuce, tomato, mayonnaise, salt, pepper, paprika, and olives (1 black).

Preparation:
-Cook the bacon in a frying pan over medium heat until crisp, then drain on a paper towel and set aside either on a plate or in the frying pan
-Cut the cooked chicken breast into thin strips no longer than one inch and set aside.
-Place the lettuce, tomatoes, green onion and bacon in a bowl. mix well with mayonnaise but do not make it too creamy
-Add salt, pepper, paprika and olives to taste.
-Top with the sliced chicken breast, and enjoy!

DINNER: **American Grilled Cheese**

Prep Time: 10 mins
Cook Time: 10 mins
Ingredients: cheddar cheese (2 slices), Monterey Jack cheese (2 slices), butter (1 tablespoon), white bread, whole wheat bread, honey (1 tablespoon)

Preparation:

-Preheat the oven to 350 degrees Fahrenheit. Butter one side of each slice of bread and place them buttered side down on the baking sheet or griddle large enough to hold all of the ingredients to be grilled, then butter the opposite side of each slice. place a slice of cheddar cheese and Monterey Jack cheese on each piece
-Grill in the oven for about 10 minutes or until the cheese is melted and bubbly
-Drizzle with some honey while they are still hot, and enjoy!

DAY 10

BREAKFAST: **American Banana Pancakes**

Prep Time: 5 mins
Cook Time: 10 mins

Ingredients: pancakes, butter, strawberry jam, bananas (2 large), orange juice (¼ cup), syrup, sugar, vanilla extract, salt, eggs (2 large), cinnamon, nutmeg.

Preparation:
-In a medium-sized bowl, whisk together two eggs, orange juice, salt, sugar and vanilla extract. add in one cup of flour
-Mix in some cinnamon and nutmeg to taste then. set aside
-Melt the butter in a frying pan on low heat and wait for it to froth but not brown. Pour about ¼ cup of batter into the frying pan allowing the batter to spread itself around then. cooking until the edges start to brown and bubbly
-Meanwhile, chop the bananas and strawberries, then layer half of them in a separate dish. Add a tablespoon or two of strawberry jam and ¼ cup of orange juice. Top with another slice of banana
-In a second frying pan, pour some batter into the centre, and cook on low heat until it is browned and bubbly.
-Top with more strawberries, jam, orange juice and bananas
-Enjoy!

LUNCH: **Turkey Ranch Wrap**

Prep Time: 10 mins
Cook Time: 10 mins

Ingredients: turkey breast (2 slices), lettuce, cheese (1 slice), cream cheese (1 tablespoon), ranch dressing, tortilla wrap.

Preparation:
-Spread about a tablespoon of cream cheese onto the tortilla spread. Add some shredded cheese and lettuce, then layer on the turkey slices and ranch dressing to taste
-Fold in the left and right sides, roll up and enjoy!

DINNER: **Chicken and Carrots**

Prep Time: 10 mins
Cook Time: 30 mins

Ingredients: chicken (1.5 pounds), carrots (2 large), olive oil, salt, pepper, rosemary, thyme, garlic powder, onions (1 large), lemon juice (½ cup), honey (1 tablespoon), parsley, parsley root, sherry wine vinegar (¼ cup).

Preparation:
-Preheat the oven to 350 degrees Fahrenheit. Coat the baking dish with olive oil and place the chicken in it. Place the baking dish in the preheated oven then. cook for about 15 minutes or until the juices run clear and the meat is almost completely cooked
-Meanwhile, scrub the parsley root to clean it then. peel and cut into small pieces or use a food processor to make them small enough
-Peel, slice and chop the carrots. Heat some olive oil in a clean pan and sauté the carrots over medium heat for about five minutes. Add in the chopped parsley root and onions. Season with salt, pepper, rosemary and thyme then. continue to cook for another five minutes
-Pour in the lemon juice and honey while still hot. Cook for a few more minutes, then pour in the sherry and parsley vinegar while still hot
-Remove the chicken from the oven, then season with salt and pepper. Serve over the carrots, garnish with fresh parsley leaves and enjoy!

DAY 11

BREAKFAST: Grilled Eggplant

Prep Time: 5 mins
Cook Time: 15 mins

Ingredients: eggplant (1 large), olive oil, salt, and black pepper, red onion (1 small), garlic powder, oregano, basil leaves, parmesan cheese (1 tablespoon), tomatoes (1 small), black olives (1 large).

Preparation:
-Slice the eggplant into slices about ½ inch thick then. coat with some salt
-In a clean frying pan, add some olive oil and wait for it to heat. Add in the eggplant slices and cook for about five minutes on each side or until browned and tender
-Peel, slice and chop the tomatoes then. chop up the olives
-Slice up the onion into small pieces or roughly chop it
-In a separate bowl, mix all the ingredients from the tomatoes, onion, olives and parmesan cheese. add a little garlic powder, oregano and fresh basil in
-Top the eggplant with the tomato mixture, and enjoy!

LUNCH: Spicy Grilled Tuna Sandwiches

Prep Time: 15 mins
Cook Time: 25 mins

Ingredients: Tuna (1 can), mayonnaise (1 tablespoon), yellow mustard (1 teaspoon), salt, pepper, lemon juice (2 tablespoons), lime juice (4 tablespoons), hot sauce (1 teaspoon), cilantro leaves, bell peppers (½ small red and ½ small green), avocado slices, lettuce, buns, tomato slices, green onion slices, black olives slices refrigerator pickles, carrot slices.

Preparation:
-Combine the avocado, lemon and lime juice in a blender or food processor, then purée until smooth
-Season with salt, pepper and hot sauce to taste, then set aside. -Drain the tuna and pat dry with paper towels. mix with some mayonnaise, yellow mustard, salt and pepper; add in plenty of cilantro leaves
-Slice the bell peppers into small pieces or cubes (for faster cooking). Slice the green onions into small pieces and slice or chop up some black olives
-Place some lettuce on the bottom buns, and also place it on the tuna sandwich. Layer with avocado slices, followed by bell peppers and some carrot slices.
-Finish with tomato slices, onion slices and some pickles sliced as well
-Enjoy!

DINNER: **Cauliflower Cheese Casserole**

Prep Time: 15 mins
Cook Time: 40 mins

Ingredients: cauliflower (1 head), olive oil, cheddar cheese (2 cups), salt, pepper, cayenne pepper, hot sauce (½ teaspoon), eggs (2 large), whole milk (½ cup), white flour (1 cup), peppercorn seasonings, butter, baking dish, plastic wrap or cooking parchment paper.

Preparation:
-Preheat the oven to 350 degrees Fahrenheit, then coat the baking dish with olive oil and set aside
-Wash the cauliflower and break it into florets in a large bowl. Toss in some salt, pepper, cayenne pepper, hot sauce and cayenne pepper to taste then. toss again lightly
-Cook the eggs over medium heat until they are soft enough then. let cool completely
-Pour a little olive oil into a clean pan on low heat, then coat the cauliflower florets add thinly sliced peppercorn seasonings -Add in the eggs, whole milk and flour then. season with salt and pepper to taste -Cook for a few minutes until the cauliflower is tender and let cool completely then. pour everything into a large mixing bowl
-Pour the cauliflower mixture into the prepared baking dish then. top with grated cheese (about ¼ cup). -Preheat the oven on high heat and place the baking dish in the oven for about 10 seconds to slightly brown the top -Place under a cooked rack for about five minutes until your cheese gets golden and melted
-Enjoy!

DAY 12

BREAKFAST: **Protein Smoothie with banana**

Prep Time: 10 mins
Cook Time: 10 mins

Ingredients: 1/2 cup egg whites (1), 1/2 cup Greek yoghurt (1), 1 cup vanilla plant milk (1), two frozen bananas (1), ice cold water (¼ cup), a pinch of cinnamon, pinch of nutmeg, hemp protein powder, flaxseed meal (½ tablespoon), cacao powder blend, ground flax seeds, a dash of vanilla extract, a tiny bit of stevia drops to taste, frozen berries (strawberries, blueberries, or blackberries), frozen spinach.

Preparation:
-Add all of the ingredients in a blender and blend until smooth
-Pour into a glass and enjoy!

LUNCH: Low Carb Chicken Breast with Roasted Asparagus

Prep Time: 15 mins
Cook Time: 35 mins

Ingredients: 3 boneless, skinless chicken breasts (1), olive oil, sage leaves, salt pepper, garlic powder, roasted asparagus spears (3 stalks), olive oil (about ¼ cup), salt and pepper to taste, lemon juice pinch of red pepper flakes for an extra kick

Preparation:
-Place the asparagus on a baking sheet lined with parchment paper, then drizzle with some olive oil and sprinkle with some salt and pepper to taste -Bake in the preheated oven at 400 degrees Fahrenheit for about 20 minutes until tender but still crunchy. Sprinkle with some more salt and pepper to taste -Sprinkle the chicken breasts with salt, black pepper and minced garlic. cook on a hot grill or pan for about 8 minutes on each side or until cooked through -Serve over the roasted asparagus
-Enjoy!

DINNER: Salmon Cakes with Avocado Dip and Healthy Coleslaw Salad

Prep Time: 10 mins
Cook Time: 40 mins

Ingredients: 2 (6 oz.) cans of salmon (1). egg whites (2 large), diced vegetables (1 cup), canned white beans (1/4 cup), olive oil, lemon juice, low sugar ketchup (½ cup), dark roast coffee instead of ketchup if you want to keep it low carb

Preparation:
-Mix egg whites and some lemon juice in a small bowl, then shape into patties and coat them with an egg wash. Bake at 350 degrees Fahrenheit for about 20 minutes until the internal temperature reaches 160 degrees Fahrenheit -In a separate bowl, mix some olive oil, ketchup, white beans, and some salt and pepper to taste. Dice up your vegetables and add them in. Mash lightly with a fork until everything is well combined -Place the mixture in a hot pan on medium heat and cook until the patties are done (about 5-8 minutes on each side)
-Finish by adding some chopped fresh parsley for colour. You can also top your salmon cakes with sautéed vegetables if you want to keep it healthier
-Serve and enjoy

DAY 13

BREAKFAST: Cinnamon French Toast with Mixed Berries and Red Pepper Cream Sauce

Prep Time: 15 mins
Cook Time: 30 mins

Ingredients: whole wheat bread (2 slices), egg whites (2 large), unsweetened almond milk (1 cup plus two tablespoons), cinnamon powder, vanilla extract, stevia drops, frozen strawberries (½ cup), frozen blueberries (½ cup), almond milk (1 teaspoon for the sauce), raspberries (1 cup).

Preparation:
-Mix the egg whites and some vanilla extract, cinnamon powder, stevia drops and almond milk in a large bowl. Dip the bread slices in the mixture until both sides are well coated. Lay them down on a baking sheet lined with parchment paper
-Bake at 375 degrees Fahrenheit for about 10 minutes or until golden browned. Flip each slice over and bake again for another 5 minutes or until golden browned again
-While the French toast is baking, mix some frozen berries, almond milk and stevia drops in a blender, then pour into a small bowl.
-Serve the French toast with some almond milk and raspberries
-Enjoy!

LUNCH: Low Carb Taco Salad with Steamed Broccoli and Low Carb Tortilla Chips

Prep Time: 15 mins
Cook Time: 25 mins

Ingredients: 1 cup low-carb tortilla chips (½ bag), black beans (1 can), tomatoes (2), diced red onion (1/8 of a large onion), chopped cilantro leaves, cheddar cheese (2 oz.), tomato sauce (½ cup), sour cream (1 tablespoon), salsa (1 teaspoon), roasted almonds, minced garlic powder, steamed broccoli florets, lime

Preparation:
-Place the broccoli florets in a pan. Add water, salt and pepper to taste then. place in a steamer for about 10 minutes or until al dente
-Meanwhile, mix the salsa and sour cream in a small bowl. Place tortilla chips and salsa sauce in a small microwave dish. cover with a lid and microwave for about one minute if you want to make them extra crispy

-Mix tomatoes, onion, cilantro leaves, and tortilla chips in a large bowl. Sprinkle some garlic powder over it for an extra kick -Serve the salad with black beans over the steamed broccoli florets. Top with cheddar cheese and add fresh lime juice
-Enjoy!

DINNER: Grilled Pork Loin with Roasted Brussels Sprouts and Creamy Pesto Sauce

Prep Time: 20 mins
Cook Time: 35 mins

Ingredients: 4 boneless pork loin chops (1 lb.), garlic powder, salt pepper to taste, one bag of frozen brussels sprouts (about one lb. or two bags of fresh sprouts), olive oil, black pepper cream cheese (4 tablespoons), basil pesto (½ cup) flaxseed meal (2 tablespoons), grated parmesan cheese (1 tablespoon), lemon juice.

Preparation:
-Mix the pesto and cream cheese in a small bowl then. set aside
-Sprinkle some salt and pepper over the pork loin chops, then place them in a hot grill pan or grill then. cook for about 5 minutes on each side or until cooked through -Move the pork chops to a serving platter. Cover with some grated cheese, then top it with a spoonful of cream cheese. spread about one tablespoon of the pesto sauce over each pork chop -Serve with roasted Brussels sprouts. Sprinkle them with some lemon juice, black pepper and flaxseed meal
-Enjoy!

DAY 14

BREAKFAST: Bacon and Egg Avocado Wrap   with Sautéed Spinach

Prep Time: 5 mins
Cook Time: 15 mins

Ingredients: 2 Bacon slices and 3 eggs (2 pieces of bacon and 3 large eggs), avocado (1), spinach (a handful), low-carb tortilla/wraps or cabbage leaves/tortillas (1), olive oil, ground black pepper, salt, lemon juice for seasoning the eggs

Preparation:
-Cook the bacon in a pan on medium to low heat until lightly crisp, then set aside on a paper towel to soak up oil and grease. crumble if desired, then set aside

-In a nonstick pan, whisk together the eggs until well blended—season with a pinch of salt and pepper.
-Place the spinach on a flat pan then. Cover with olive oil and add salt to taste. Cook for about 1 or 2 minutes
-On each tortilla/wrap, mix 1/2 sliced avocado, eggs, and bacon crumbles, then wrap it in some cabbage leaves or other tortilla/wrap as desired
-Serve with some lemon juice to season the eggs
-Enjoy!

LUNCH: **Crab Cakes with Low Carb Caesar Salad and Blue Cheese Dressing or Mayonnaise**

Prep Time: 20 mins
Cook Time: 25 mins

Ingredients: 1 small can of crab meat (½ cup), two organic eggs, two tablespoons of shredded Parmesan cheese (1 oz.), ½ tablespoon of dried parsley leaves, one clove of garlic, minced and de-skinned, 1/4 teaspoon of salt (or to taste) ½ tablespoon coconut oil for frying, sliced olives for garnish if desired

Preparation:
-In a large bowl, mix the eggs, sea salt, black pepper and coconut oil, then add the rest of the ingredients until well blended.
-Add the crab meat and mix well then. let the mixture sit for about 15 minutes to let the ingredients meld
-Preheat a skillet on medium to low heat, then add enough oil to coat the pan. Flatten out the mixture into about 1-inch-thick patties. fry for about 2 or 3 minutes on each side, turning once
-Serve with a side salad and blue cheese dressing/mayonnaise over the top or with a side of your choice
-Enjoy!

DINNER: **Baked Salmon with Stuffed Peppers and Carrot Salad**

Prep Time: 15 mins
Cook Time: 45 mins

Ingredients: 1 can of salmon (6 oz.) ½ red onion, thinly sliced. 2 cups chopped mushrooms, 1 cup grated zucchini (1 zucchini), ½ cup shredded carrots, 3 chopped green onions or chives, ½ teaspoon garlic powder or minced garlic cloves, 1 teaspoon ground black pepper. ½ cup almond flour (3 tablespoons), 1 or 2 teaspoons of olive oil for the salmon, 2 bell peppers, seeded and de-seeded roasted almonds, chopped chives or parsley for garnish if desired

Preparation:
-Preheat the oven to 350 °F
-In a medium bowl, mix the red onion, green onion/chives and garlic cloves until well blended, then add some pepper and salt to taste and set aside
-Add some olive oil to a hot skillet over medium heat, then add the chopped mushrooms until golden brown. Add the carrots, zucchini and sliced peppers, garlic powder and black pepper
-Spoon about 1/3 cup of the mixture into a small bowl. Spoon out some salmon into the middle of the mixture. Roll into a ball and place in the skillet. Add in some almond flour. If the mixture is wetter than desired, add more flour
-Cook for about 5 minutes or until the salmon is cooked through, then serve with lemon wedges and carrot salad on the side
-Enjoy!

DAY 15

BREAKFAST: **Eggs Benedict with Savory Ham English Muffin and Hollandaise Sauce**

Prep Time: 5 mins
Cook Time: 10 mins

Ingredients: 1 slice of ham, 2 slices of fully cooked egg, 1 leaf of spinach, 4 slices low carb bread (1 slice for each bread), hollandaise sauce (2 tablespoons), lemon juice

Preparation:
-In a small bowl, mix the hollandaise sauce then. set aside -Place each slice of bread in a pan then. grill them on medium to low heat until lightly toasted on both sides and cooked through on the inside
-In a nonstick pan, lightly sauté the spinach and ham with some salt, pepper and lemon juice until the spinach is wilted. Transfer to serving plates or place on top of bread slices as desired -Place one slice

of bread on each plate then. Place an egg over the bread slice, cover the egg with another slice of bread as desired -Drizzle some hollandaise sauce over the bread and eggs and top it off with a piece of ham. Serve with a side salad if desired
-Enjoy!

LUNCH: **Savory Chicken and Almond Butter Sandwich**

Prep Time: 15 mins
Cook Time: 20 mins

Ingredients: 1 tablespoon creamy or chunky almond butter, 2 slices low carb naan or savory bread (1 slice for each sandwich), chicken breast (2), 1 small avocado, spring onions/scallions, sliced olives, sea salt, ground black pepper and lemon juice for seasoning the chicken.

Preparation:

-In a bowl, mix the almond butter and chicken with some pepper and sea salt to taste and set aside
-In another medium bowl, mix the sliced olives, minced onions/scallions, garlic powder and olive oil and set aside -Heat a pan on medium to low heat. Add in the chicken breast, pepper, sea salt, and lemon juice. Cook the chicken for about 6 to 10 minutes or until the chicken is thoroughly cooked through then. set aside -Add some olive oil to a skillet over medium heat, then layer out slices of naan or bread seasoned with pepper and sea salt as desired -Place an egg omelette in the middle of each naan/bread slice. Top it off with sliced avocado, almond butter chicken, spring onions/scallions' mixture and olives -Serve with lemon wedges on top, and enjoy!

DINNER: **Roasted Salmon with Green Beans or a Side Salad**

Prep Time: 15 mins
Cook Time: 35 mins

Ingredients: 2 pieces of salmon, 1 tablespoon of olive oil for roasting, sea salt and ground black pepper for seasoning the salmon (to taste), 1 stalk of celery, cut into ribbons, 1 cup green beans, trimmed and cut into 2-inch by ½ inch pieces, 2 tablespoons minced parsley leaves, 1 tablespoon minced onion, 1 teaspoon sea salt. ¼ teaspoon pepper (or to taste)

Preparation:

-In a small bowl, add some olive oil—season with sea salt and pepper to taste. Mix well, then rub the oil over the skin of the salmon until fully coated on all sides. Set the smoked salmon aside to marinate for about 15 minutes. -Add some olive oil to a skillet over medium heat. Add in the celery and sauté for about 2 minutes until slightly crispy and slightly browned
-Add in the green beans and season with sea salt and pepper. Cook until tender, then transfer beans to the serving plate or bowl -Add some more olive oil to a skillet over medium heat. Add in some fish

if desired, season with sea salt, ground black pepper, and saute until cooked through while turning often. serve with the celery and green beans
-Enjoy!

DAY 16

BREAKFAST: Ham and Cheese Egg Muffin Cups

Prep Time: 10 mins
Cook Time: 30 mins

Ingredients: 2 large eggs. 1 sliced ham. 1 sliced cheese. 2 slices low carb bread (1 slice for each muffin). ½ teaspoon dried parsley leaves. salt and ground black pepper to taste (or to taste)

Preparation:
-Preheat the oven to 400°F, then line a baking sheet with foil. Coat foil with some oil. Place each slice of bread on the baking sheet and spray some oil over them. Bake for about 8 minutes or until lightly toasted around the edges. Remove from the oven and set aside.
-In a small bowl, mix the eggs, ham, parsley, salt and pepper until well blended. Scoop out about 1/3 cup of the mixture into a small muffin cup. Add in each slice of cheese over the top as desired -Add some more oil to a skillet over medium heat. Add in the eggs and cook until slightly firm, about 2 minutes and set aside
 -Add some more oil to a skillet over medium to low heat. Place one bread slice over on top. Add the eggs on top and place another bread slice on it, so it covers the eggs completely -Place another muffin tin on top of the first one. bake for about 30 minutes or until firm when pressed lightly with your finger (or toasted lightly)
-Enjoy!

LUNCH: Savory Fish eggy Sandwich

Prep Time: 15 mins
Cook Time: 25 mins

Ingredients: 2 tablespoons creamy or chunky almond butter (1 tablespoon), 2 slices half slice low carb bread (1 slice for each sandwich), 2 ounces salmon, 2 slices red onion, thinly sliced, 2 ounces canned tuna in water, 1 tablespoon minced parsley leaves, 1 teaspoon minced garlic (or to taste), 1 tablespoon lemon juice

Preparation:

-In a small bowl, mix the almond butter, parsley, garlic and lemon juice and set aside
-Spread some oil over a nonstick pan. Place the slices of salmon and onion on top of the pan and season with sea salt and ground black pepper to taste then. cook on medium to low heat for about 3 minutes on each side (or until grilled)
-Drizzle about one tablespoon of the almond butter mixture over one slice of bread. Place the salmon and onion slices in the middle. Place a slice of tuna on top. cover with another slice of bread as desired
-Place an egg in the middle of each sandwich then. Cover with a piece of bread. Drizzle some more almond butter mixture over the sandwiches.
-Squeeze some lemon wedges over each one while it is still warm, and enjoy!
-Note: Add a slice of cucumber or lettuce to the sandwich if desired.

DINNER: **Mashed Cauliflower**

Prep Time: 15 mins
Cook Time: 25 mins

Ingredients: 1 tablespoon unsalted butter or ghee. 1 tablespoon almond milk or cream. 2 cloves garlic, minced (or to taste). 1/2 small head of cauliflower, cut into florets (about 4 cups). sea salt and ground black pepper to taste (or to taste)

Preparation:

-Place 1 tablespoon of butter on top of a skillet over medium heat. Add in the garlic, then season with sea salt and pepper to taste. Saute for about 2 minutes then.
-Add cauliflower florets, sea salt and pepper (to taste).
Frequently stir while cooking until cauliflower is fork tender
-Transfer to a bowl and serve while warm over top of some mashed potatoes!

DAY 17

BREAKFAST: **Baked Eggs with Avocado & Tomato**

Prep Time: 5 mins
Cook Time: 15 mins

Ingredients: 2 large eggs (or 4 small), 1/4 medium or small avocado (or 1 slice deli turkey), 2 cubes of mozzarella cheese, 1 tomato, 2 tablespoons chopped fresh cilantro leaves, salt and ground black pepper to taste

Preparation:
-Mix the eggs, avocado, mozzarella cheese, and cilantro in a bowl. Season with sea salt and pepper to taste. Spoon into a small baking dish. Add some oil on top of the egg mixture. Bake at 400° F for about 12 minutes or until firm and slightly toasted around the edges
-Enjoy!

LUNCH: Baked Salmon with Spinach & Pineapple

Prep Time: 15 mins
Cook Time: 35 mins

Ingredients: 1 cup baby spinach leaves. 1 cup fresh, chopped strawberries. 2 ounces canned salmon (or canned smoked salmon), 1 tablespoon coconut oil, 1/2 medium red onion, 1/2 medium green bell pepper, 3 cubes of chicken broth (1 cube for each can of salmon), 2 teaspoons lemon juice (optional), sea salt and ground black pepper to taste, a pinch of turmeric

Preparation:
-Place coconut oil in a small skillet over low heat. Add onion and red bell pepper and sauté until tender while stirring frequently. Season with sea salt and pepper to taste. turn off the heat and set aside
-Preheat the oven at 400° F then. place the spinach leaves in a baking dish
-Add in some oil over a large skillet over medium heat, then place the salmon in the large skillet and cook on both sides until lightly browned. Remove from the oven and set aside
-In a small bowl, mix the coconut oil and spinach leaves (season with sea salt and pepper to taste. Spoon over the salmon and mix. add in the sliced pineapple, chicken broth and lemon juice
-Arrange the spinach on top of each serving plate. Place a scoop of the salmon over the spinach, then drizzle with the pineapple mixture
-Top with some additional pineapple, and enjoy!

DINNER: Chicken Fajita

Prep Time: 15 mins
Cook Time: 25 mins

Ingredients: 2 chicken thighs (or breasts), boneless and skinless. 1 tablespoon olive oil, 1/2 medium red onion, thinly sliced, 2 garlic cloves, minced or pressed (or to taste), 1 teaspoon ground cumin, 1

teaspoon ground coriander (or to taste), a pinch of sea salt and ground black pepper, a pinch of cayenne pepper
-Preheat the oven to 400°F. Coat a shallow baking dish with olive oil or spray with nonstick cooking spray. Place the chicken in the baking dish then. bake for about 20 minutes or until lightly browned
-While the chicken is baking, place a skillet over medium heat. Add in one teaspoon of olive oil, then add onion and garlic and season with sea salt and pepper to taste. sauté for about 2 minutes then. Add in the ground cumin, coriander and cayenne. sauté for about 1 minute. Add in the marinade (from chicken), then cook for about 3 minutes or until onions are tender
-Place the cooked chicken on top of the onions. Spoon the onions over top of the chicken and serve while warm
-Enjoy!

DAY 18

BREAKFAST: Ricotta and Honey Toast with Fresh Fruit
Prep Time: 5 mins
Cook Time: 10 mins

Ingredients: 1 slice of bread, 1 tablespoon ricotta cheese (or to taste), 2 tablespoons honey, 2 tablespoons shredded Parmesan cheese (or 1 tablespoon slivered almonds (optional)

Preparation:
-Preheat the oven to 400°F. Place a baking sheet on the middle rack of the oven to preheat then.
-In a small bowl, mix ricotta cheese and honey until well combined
-Spread ricotta and honey over one slice of bread, sprinkle with Parmesan cheese. Top with almonds if desired
-Place bread slice on top of a baking sheet. Bake for 8 minutes or until the edges turn golden brown
-Enjoy!

LUNCH: Creamy Potato Soup with Cheddar and Chives
Prep Time: 15 mins
Cook Time: 20 mins

Ingredients: 1 cup peeled and diced potatoes (or other vegetables -optional) 3 cups vegetable broth, 1/2 cup light cream, 1 tablespoon minced onion (or to taste), 2 tablespoons flour (or to taste), 1 tablespoon olive oil (or to taste), 1/2 teaspoon salt, pepper to taste.

Preparation:

-Place a large pot on stovetop over medium heat. Add in some oil then add in the diced potatoes. Cook for about 10 minutes or until tender. Add in the rest of your ingredients and season with sea salt and pepper to taste. Cover with a lid and cook for 20 minutes (resting time)
-Transfer to a bowl, add more pepper and salt to taste if desired
-Enjoy!

DINNER: Roasted Brussels Sprouts with Balsamic Vinegar

Prep Time: 10 mins
Cook Time: 30 mins

Ingredients: 1 pound Brussels sprouts, cut into ½ inch slices, 2 tablespoons olive oil, salt to taste, 1/2 teaspoon black pepper

Preparation:

-Preheat the oven to 400°F. In a large bowl, toss the Brussels sprouts in EVOO (or olive oil) then spread on cookie sheets lined with parchment paper or nonstick foil. Season with sea salt and pepper to taste. Roast for about 25 minutes or until tender -While the Brussels sprouts are roasting, mix the balsamic vinegar together with some olive oil, salt and pepper in a small bowl. Place the roasted Brussels sprouts in a serving bowl and drizzle with balsamic vinegar mixture
-Enjoy!

DAY 19

BREAKFAST: Peanut Butter Banana Oatmeal

Prep Time: 10 mins *
Cook Time: 30 mins

Ingredients: 1 cup plain, nonfat yogurt (or coconut milk) 3/4 teaspoon pure vanilla extract, 1/2 medium banana, mashed (or frozen banana for thickening, optional), 1 cup cooked steel cut oats, milk to desired consistency.

Preparation:

-Place all of the ingredients in a small saucepan over low heat or microwave. Mix well -Lastly, add in the chopped peanuts -Enjoy!

LUNCH: Broccoli Cheddar Soup

Prep Time: 10 mins
Cook Time: 20 mins

Ingredients: 8 ounces broccoli florets (fresh), 1 cup fat free milk, 1/2 cup shredded Cheddar cheese (or mozzarella), 2 tablespoons all-purpose flour, 1 teaspoon butter, 1/2 teaspoons salt (or to taste) ground black pepper to taste, cooking spray (or a small amount of butter)

Preparation:

In a small saucepan over medium heat, melt butter then add flour until well incorporated. Add in the milk and season with sea salt and pepper to taste. Whisk until smooth then add in the cheese. Stir through then add in the broccoli florets to the saucepan. Reduce heat and cook for about 7 minutes or until thoroughly heated through. -Transfer to a small bowl and serve immediately while warm.

DINNER: Steamed Broccoli with Garlic & Olive Oil

Prep Time: 5 mins
Cook Time: 10 mins

Ingredients: 1/2 medium head of broccoli, cut into bite-size pieces, 2 cloves garlic finely chopped, 1 tablespoon olive oil, cooking spray or a small amount of butter, salt and pepper to taste.

Preparation:
Place a steamer basket in a large pot with enough water to cover the bottom, then turn the heat to high. When the water comes to a boil, add in broccoli florets, then cover and cook for about 3 minutes or until tender-crisp then remove it from heat and drain well. -In a small bowl combine garlic, olive oil, sea salt and pepper to taste.
-Place broccoli into a large bowl and drizzle with olive oil mixture. Sprinkle with sea salt and pepper to taste. Serve immediately.
-Enjoy!

DAY 20

BREAKFAST: Chocolate Chip Waffles

Prep Time: 30 mins
Cook Time: 15 mins

Ingredients: 6 eggs, 1/2 cup pumpkin puree (or pure maple syrup, 1 teaspoon vanilla extract), 1/4 cup olive oil (or coconut oil), 1/3 cup packed, brown sugar (plus extra for serving), 2 cups whole-wheat flour (plus extra for serving) 2 teaspoons baking powder, 1/2 teaspoon salt, 3 tablespoons cocoa powder or cacao nibs.

Preparation: -Preheat oven to 350°F. Place a cast iron skillet on stove top over medium heat, add some olive oil, and place the waffle iron inside.
-Add some water to the waffle iron, then add all your ingredients. Mix well then place in oven for about 15 minutes or until golden brown.
-Transfer to a serving dish, add more sea salt and cocoa powder to taste if desired, then serve with extra cocoa powder.
-Enjoy!

LUNCH: Carrot Ginger Soup

Prep Time: 10 mins
Cook Time: 45 mins

Ingredients: 2 tablespoons butter, 5 carrots, peeled and sliced, 1/2 cup chopped onions (or shallots if preferred), 1/2 teaspoon sea salt (or to taste) 5 cups chicken broth, 3 tablespoons ginger root, finely grated, 2 tablespoons lemon juice, freshly ground black pepper to taste, Pinch of cayenne pepper or red pepper flakes.

Preparation:
-Melt the butter in a large saucepan over medium heat. Add onions, carrots and sea salt and cook for 15 minutes or until tender. Pour the chicken broth into the saucepan, then add ginger, cayenne and lemon juice. Bring it to a boil, then reduce heat to low simmer for about 30 minutes or until carrots are tender.
-Transfer to a blender or food processor and blend until smooth. Stir through until well combined. Serve with additional sea salt and pepper if desired.
-Enjoy!

DINNER: **Green Beans Almondine or Amandine**

Prep Time: 10 mins
Cook Time: 20 mins

Ingredients: 1 tablespoon butter, 1 cup shiitake mushrooms, sliced, 1 cup green beans (fresh), 1/2 teaspoon sea salt (or to taste), 1/2 teaspoon freshly ground black pepper (to taste), Cooking spray or butter for greasing (for thickening the sauce), 2 tablespoons almond meal (or almond flour)

Preparation:

-In a large pot over high heat, add some extra virgin olive oil then butter. Place the sauté pan on the stovetop over medium heat, then add mushrooms, sea salt, and pepper to taste. Stir through until the mushrooms have softened and browned well.
-Add in the green beans then cook for about 2-3 minutes or until tender-crisp. Toss through in the mushrooms, then add in the almond meal (if using). Whisk through until combined then smooth out with a whisk. Return to a low simmer, then transfer to a blender or food processor and blend until smooth. Pour back into the pot over medium heat and cook for about 15 minutes or until thickened up slightly. Season with additional sea salt and pepper if desired. Stir through until well combined and serve immediately.
-Enjoy!

DAY 21

BREAKFAST: **Cinnamon Rolls**

Prep Time: 15 mins
Cook Time: 20 mins

Ingredients: 2 1/2 cups all-purpose flour, 1 tablespoon baking powder, 1/4 cup packed brown sugar, 1 tablespoon cinnamon (plus more for sprinkling), 1 teaspoon ground nutmeg, 3 eggs.

Preparation:

-Mix all of the ingredients then add in more if needed. Pour into a deep greased pan, then cook in the oven for about 20 minutes or until golden brown and cooked through. Serve immediately with butter and orange marmalade on the side.
-Enjoy!

LUNCH: **Roasted Butternut Squash Soup**

Prep Time: 15 mins
Cook Time: 1 hour

Ingredients: 2 pounds butternut squash, 1 large yellow onion, chopped, 2 tablespoons extra-virgin olive oil, 8 cups vegetable broth or chicken broth, 1/2 teaspoon ground cinnamon (or more to taste), Sea salt and freshly ground black pepper to taste, 3 tablespoons butter or cream if desired.

Preparation:
Peel and seed butternut squash then cut into small cubes. Place on a parchment-lined baking sheet, then toss through in olive oil, sea salt and pepper. Bake in oven at 400°F for about 20-25 minutes or until fork tender. Prepare the soup base by heating oil in a large saucepan over medium high heat. Cook onions for about 5 minutes or until tender, add in vegetable broth, then cinnamon. Bring to a boil, then reduce heat to low simmer for about 45 minutes or until onions are tender. Add squash and cook for another 5 minutes or so until soft and tender.
-Transfer blender then blend into a smooth puree while adding the butter (if using) gradually through the center hole of the lid. Season with additional sea salt and pepper if desired.
-Enjoy!

DINNER: **Sautéed Kale**

Prep Time: 5 mins
Cook Time: 10 mins

Ingredients: 1 bunch kale, 1 tablespoon extra-virgin olive oil (or more if desired), Sea salt and freshly ground black pepper to taste, freshly grated Parmesan cheese for topping,

Preparation:
Wash, then prepare the kale by removing the leaves from the stem and tearing them into smaller pieces. Place in a large bowl, add in sea salt, black pepper and olive oil then massage into the kale until well coated. Heat some extra virgin olive oil in a frying pan over medium heat then place kale in the pan so that it's covering it well. Preheat oven to 350 degrees F (175 degrees C) and brush an ovenproof dish with oil. Pour the cornbread batter into the dish, bake for 25 minutes or until firm.
-In a large frying pan over medium heat, add some extra virgin olive oil then sauté pine nuts and garlic until golden brown.
-Add in kale then reduce heat to low simmer for about 5 minutes or until kale is tender, continue cooking until some liquid has evaporated out of the pan. Season with additional sea salt, pepper and Parmesan cheese if desired.
-Serve immediately topped with Parmesan cheese.
-Enjoy!

DAY 22

BREAKFAST: Orange Cranberry Muffins

Prep Time: 15 mins
Cook Time: 25 mins

Ingredients: 1/2 cup butter, (1 stick), 1 cup brown sugar, 3 eggs (beaten), 1 teaspoon vanilla extract, 2 cups all-purpose flour, 1 teaspoon baking powder, 3 teaspoons orange zest (plus more for sprinkling on muffins).

Preparation:

-Preheat oven to 350 degrees F (175 degrees C) then grease a muffin tray well. In a large bowl, add butter and brown sugar, then cream until combined well. Add in eggs one at a time beating well after each addition until blended.
-In a small bowl, sift in flour, flour, baking powder, baking soda, salt and orange zest. Combine well then spoon into butter mixture then mix until combined. Fold through dried cranberries, whole cranberries and orange juice until well combined.
-Spoon batter evenly into the muffin tray and sprinkle with more orange zest if desired or leave plain. Bake for about 20 minutes or until a skewer inserted into the center of the muffins come out clean.
-Enjoy!

LUNCH: Cream of Tomato Soup

Prep Time: 20 mins
Cook Time: 30 mins

Ingredients: 2 tablespoons extra virgin olive oil, 1 medium onion, 4 cloves garlic, 3 tablespoons flour, 1 tablespoon dried oregano (plus more for seasoning), 2 cans (14.7 ounces each) fire-roasted diced tomatoes with juice, 1 can (12 ounces) vegetable stock or water.

Preparation:

-Heat oil in a deep saucepan over medium heat, then add in onions and garlic and cook until soft and translucent. Add in flour to the onion and garlic mixture, stir until combined well, then add in tomatoes and vegetable stock or water. Stir through and bring to a boil. Reduce heat to low simmer for about 30 minutes or until thickened up slightly. Season with additional oregano if desired.
-Serve immediately.
-Enjoy!

DINNER: Cauliflower "Rice" Pilaf

Prep Time: 15 mins
Cook Time: 30 mins

Ingredients: 1 cup cauliflower florets, 1 medium yellow onion, 1/2 inch chopped, 3 cloves garlic (plus more for sautéing), 2 tablespoons butter or olive oil, 2 cups vegetable stock or chicken stock.

Preparation:
-Peel and then chop cauliflower florets into bite-size pieces. Heat oil or butter in a medium saucepan over medium heat, add cauliflower and onion, and cook until tender. Add in the chopped garlic and cook for another minute.
Be careful not to overcook the cauliflower otherwise it will become soggy and fall apart. Season with sea salt and pepper, then stir and add in vegetable stock or chicken stock. Bring to a boil, then reduce heat to low simmer for about 20 minutes or until cauliflower is tender.
-Serve immediately.

DAY 23

BREAKFAST: Tropical Fruit Salad with Honey and Lime

Prep Time: 15 mins
Cook Time: 5 mins

Ingredients: 1 pineapple (cut into bite-size chunks), 1 mango (peeled, pitted and cut into bite-size chunks), 2 kiwis (peeled and sliced), 1 cup seedless grapes, 1/3 cup fresh mint leaves, 2 tablespoons honey, 1 teaspoon fresh lime juice,

Preparation:
-Combine pineapple, mango fruits and grapes in a large bowl, then add mint leaves. In a small bowl, whisk together honey and lime juice until smooth, then drizzle over fruit. Toss around to coat evenly then serve.

LUNCH: Cauliflower Soup

Prep Time: 15 mins
Cook Time: 1 hour

Ingredients: 1 medium onion, 2 tablespoons extra virgin olive oil, (1 tablespoon if desired), 2 cloves garlic, 1 head cauliflower florets, 2 teaspoons sea salt, 3 cups vegetable stock or chicken stock.

Preparation:

-Peel and then chop cauliflower into bite-size pieces. In a large saucepan, heat oil over medium heat, add onion and garlic and cook until soft and translucent. Add cauliflower pieces and sea salt to the onions, then stir and add in vegetable stock or chicken stock. Bring to a boil, then reduce heat to low simmer for about 20 minutes or until tender.
Preheat oven to 350 degrees F (175 degrees C) and line a baking sheet with parchment paper, pierce with cauliflower with a fork then place on baking sheet. Bake for 10-15 minutes or until golden brown. Place in an airtight container and refrigerate overnight.
-Serve soup chilled topped with roasted cauliflower croutons.

DINNER: Braised Red Cabbage

Prep Time: 20 mins
Cook Time: 40 mins

Ingredients: 1 medium onion, 2 tablespoons extra virgin olive oil, 1 head red cabbage, 4 cups chicken stock, 3 tablespoons red wine vinegar.

Preparation:

-Chop cabbage into bite-size pieces and set aside. Heat oil in a large saucepan over medium heat, add onions, and cook until soft. Add in cabbage to the onion mixture, then stir through and add in chicken stock, bring to a boil, then reduce heat to low simmer for about 15 minutes or until cabbage is tender.
-Transfer cabbage and onions into a large bowl, drizzle with red wine vinegar, and season with sea salt and pepper if desired. Serve immediately.

DAY 24

BREAKFAST: Yogurt Parfait with Mixed Berries and Pecans

Prep Time: 10 mins
Cook Time: 10 mins

Ingredients: 1 cup plain yogurt, 1 cup blueberries, 1/2 cup pecans.

Preparation: -In a small bowl, whisk yogurt with 1 teaspoon honey until smooth then set aside. In a medium size glass or jar, layer yogurt, add a few spoonful of blueberries, then top with pecans. -Top with a few more blueberries, pecans and drizzle with honey. Serve immediately.

LUNCH: Vegetable Beef Soup

Prep Time: 15 mins
Cook Time: 1 hour

Ingredients: 6 carrots, 1 medium yellow onion, 2 stalks celery (with leaves), 2 tablespoons extra virgin olive oil (or vegetable oil), 3 cloves garlic, 1 cup water, 3 cups beef broth or vegetable broth, salt and freshly ground black pepper (to taste)

Preparation:

-Peel carrots, yellow onion and celery then chop into bite-size pieces. Heat oil in a large saucepan over medium heat, then add in chopped vegetables and garlic and cook until soft. Add in water, beef broth or vegetable broth and then season with additional salt and pepper if desired. Bring to a boil, then reduce heat to low simmer for about 30 minutes or until vegetables are tender.
-Enjoy!

DINNER: Stir-Fried Brussels Sprouts and Asparagus with Brown Rice

Prep Time: 15 mins
Cook Time: 35 mins

Ingredients: 1 tablespoon butter or lard, 1/4 cup ground cashews. 1 1/2 pounds Brussels sprouts, ends removed, coarsely chopped (about 4 cups), 8 ounces fresh asparagus, tough ends removed and cut into 1 1/4-inch piece, 3 cups cooked brown rice.

Preparation:

-Melt butter or lard in a large saucepan over medium heat, add cashews, and cook until lightly browned. Add in Brussels sprouts and asparagus to the saucepan and cook for 4 minutes. Add in brown rice and toss around to coat evenly then reduce heat to low simmer and cook for about 5 minutes. Season with sea salt and pepper if desired.
-Serve topped with sesame seeds, sesame oil, or cashews if desired.
-Enjoy!

DAY 25

BREAKFAST: Overnight Oats with Chia Seeds and Coconut Milk

Prep Time: 10 mins
Cook Time: 5 mins

Ingredients: 3/4 cup steel-cut oats, 2 cups water, 1 1/2 teaspoons chia seeds, 1 teaspoon vanilla extract (optional), 4 tablespoons unsweetened shredded coconut flakes.

Preparation:

-In a small bowl, add steel-cut oats, water, and chia seeds, stir together, then cover and refrigerate overnight. In the morning, add coconut flakes and vanilla extract if desired, then stir. Serve cold.

LUNCH: Spicy Philly Cheese Steak

Prep Time: 10 mins
Cook Time: 15 mins

Ingredients: 1 tablespoon butter or lard, 2 tablespoons extra long grain white rice flour, 1 pound beefsteak, 1 tablespoon sea salt, 1 tablespoon brown sugar.

Preparation:

-Heat butter or lard in a large ovenproof sauté pan over medium-high flame, then add in rice flour and pork, cook until lightly browned. Cook until no longer pink and transfer to a plate, season with sea salt and brown sugar.
-Sauté onions until transparent, then add in green peppers and cook for 3 minutes.
-Add in beefsteak, sea salt and brown sugar to the pan then cook for 2 minutes on each side.
-Serve topped with chopped onions, peppers and green onions.
-Enjoy!

DINNER: **Lemon Dill Green Beans**

Prep Time: 10 mins
Cook Time: 20 mins

Ingredients: 2 cups trimmed green beans, 1 teaspoon extra virgin olive oil, 1/3 cup dry bread crumbs. 1/4 cup water, 1/4 cup minced onion, 1 clove garlic (minced), 2 tablespoons unsalted butter, 1 tablespoon olive oil, 2 sprigs of dill, 1 lemon (zested and cut into wedges).

Preparation:

-Bring a medium size pot of salted water to a boil over high heat, then add in green beans and cook for about 5 minutes or until tender but still firm. Drain from water and set aside.
-Heat extra virgin olive oil in a large saucepan over medium heat, then add in onions and garlic, and cook for about 3 minutes or until translucent. Add in butter or lard and cook for 1 minute, then add bread crumbs, water, and lemon zest. Remove from heat and toss to coat evenly.
-Combine green beans and dill with bread crumb mixture, drizzle with extra virgin olive oil, and garnish with chopped green onions if desired. Serve hot topped with lemon wedges or lemon slices.

DAY 26

BREAKFAST: **Zucchini Bread**

Prep Time: 10 mins
Cook Time: 40 mins

Ingredients: 2 1/2 cups all-purpose flour, 3/4 cup sugar, 2 teaspoons baking powder, 1/2 teaspoon baking soda, 1 teaspoon. Ground cinnamon, 1/2 teaspoon salt, 4 eggs, 1/2 cup vegetable oil, 1/2 cup applesauce, 2 teaspoons vanilla extract, 2 cups zucchini (grated and squeezed dry), 1 1/2 cups chopped pecans.

Preparation:

-Preheat oven to 350 F, then lightly grease a 5 by 9-inch loaf pan. In a large bowl, combine flour, sugar baking powder, soda, ground cinnamon, and salt mixing until blended. In another bowl, beat together eggs, vegetable oil, applesauce and vanilla extract until well blended then beat in grated zucchini and chopped pecans. Add egg mixture to flour mixture and stir until just combined. Pour batter into prepared pan then bake for 40-50 minutes or until toothpick inserted into center of loaf comes out clean. Allow to cool in pan 10 minutes then remove from pan and cool completely before slicing.

LUNCH: **Chicken Philly Cheesesteak Sandwich**
Prep Time: 5 mins
Cook Time: 15 mins

Ingredients: 1 pound ground chicken breast, 1 teaspoon dried oregano, salt and pepper, 1/4 cup olive oil, 3 ounces provolone cheese (shredded), 2 tablespoons butter, 8 slices white bread.

Preparation:
-Lightly pound ground chicken, add in oregano and salt and pepper, mix until combined, and then form into 4 patties.
-Heat olive oil and butter in a large nonstick skillet over medium heat, then add in chicken patties, cook for 6 to 8 minutes on each side. Remove from pan and set aside.
-Add back into pan provolone cheese (1 ounce per sandwich) along with 2 tablespoons butter or lard then cook for about 1 minute on each side until browned. Repeat with remaining sandwiches.
-Serve topped with shredded provolone cheese and dill pickle chips if desired.
-Enjoy!

DINNER: **Baked Salmon with Pecan Crust**
Prep Time: 10 mins
Cook Time: 25 mins

Ingredients: 4 pieces Wild Caught Sockeye Salmon, 1 teaspoon sea salt, 1/2 teaspoon ground black pepper, 1 cup all-purpose flour, 4 tablespoons butter or lard, 1 large egg white.

Preparation:
-Heat oven to 375 degrees, then lightly grease 6 individual pie dishes. In a small mixing bowl, add the salt and pepper and mix well. In a large mixing bowl, combine the salmon, flour, and egg whites, then form into 6 patties.
-Place patties into prepared pie dishes then coat each patty with the salt and pepper mixture. Add 2 tablespoons butter or lard to each pie dish then bake in preheated oven for 15-20 minutes or until golden brown.
-Serve topped with mango chutney and spinach if desired.
-Enjoy!

DAY 27

BREAKFAST: Creamy Tomato Soup

Prep Time: 15 mins
Cook Time: 20 mins

Ingredients: 1 tablespoon extra-virgin olive oil, 1/3 cup chopped onion, 2 cloves garlic (minced), 1 green bell pepper (diced), 14.5 ounces crushed tomatoes, salt and pepper to taste.

Preparation:

-Heat extra virgin olive oil in a large saucepan over medium heat, then add in onion and garlic, sauté until translucent. Add in bell peppers and tomatoes, then cook for 10 minutes or until sauce is bubbly. Season with sea salt and black pepper to taste, then puree in a blender or food processor until smooth.
-Enjoy!

LUNCH: Squash and Cheese Enchiladas

Prep Time: 10 mins
Cook Time: 30 mins

Ingredients: 2 tablespoons olive oil, 4 large eggs, 1/2 cup sour cream, 2 cups cubed butternut squash, 1 cup shredded Monterey Jack cheese, 1 teaspoon chili powder. 1 cup cheddar cheese (shredded), 8 corn tortillas (about 6 inches in diameter), 1 teaspoon sea salt.

Preparation:

-Heat olive oil in a large nonstick skillet over medium heat, then add in corn tortillas one at a time and fry until golden brown. Remove from pan and set aside. Add 1/2 tablespoon olive oil to skillet and place in the cubed squash, then cook for about 6 minutes or until tender. Remove from pan and set aside.
-Increase heat to medium-high, then add in eggs and whisk until blended then stir in sour cream, chili powder and salt. Pour 1 cup of the butternut squash mixture into each tortilla followed by 1/4 cup shredded cheeses then roll up individual enchiladas.
-Heat 2 tablespoons olive oil over medium heat in a large nonstick skillet then brown the enchiladas on all sides (about 5 minutes). Place into lightly greased baking dish and repeat with remaining tortillas. Top each dish with remaining squash mixture, then sprinkle with remaining cheeses.
-Bake in 350-degree oven for 20 minutes or until heated through.
-Enjoy!

DINNER: **Chili with Meet**

Prep Time: 15 mins
Cook Time: 35 mins

Ingredients: 2 pounds lean ground beef, 1 teaspoon ground cumin, 1 teaspoon chili powder, 2 teaspoons sugar (optional), 1 clove garlic (minced), 1 can diced tomatoes (undrained), 4 cups beef broth, 8 ounces sour cream.

Preparation:

-Heat a large Dutch oven over medium-high heat, then add in 1 tablespoon olive oil and ground beef. Cook for about 8 minutes, stirring frequently or until cooked through. Reduce heat to medium then add in cumin, chili powder and sugar if desired, garlic and cook for about 1 minute. Add in diced tomatoes with juice, beef broth and sour cream then stir to combine. Continue cooking for 15 minutes or until heated through.
-Enjoy!

DAY 28

BREAKFAST: **Roasted Butternut Squash Soup**

Prep Time: 15 mins
Cook Time: 40 mins

Ingredients: 3 cups butternut squash (peeled, seeded and cubed), 2 tablespoons olive oil, 1 medium yellow onion (diced). 4 cloves garlic (minced), 1 cup chopped celery, 4 cups chicken broth. Salt and pepper to taste.

Preparation:

-Heat oven to 350 degrees. Place butternut squash on a rimmed baking sheet then toss with olive oil then season with sea salt and black pepper. Roast in preheated oven for 20 minutes or until tender then set aside.
-Heat olive oil in a large saucepan over medium-high heat, then add in onion and garlic, sauté until translucent. Add in celery, broth, roasted butternut squash and cook for about 10 minutes or until heated through.
-Puree with an immersion blender or food processor until smooth then serve warm.
-Enjoy!

LUNCH: **Grilled Chicken or Turkey with Roasted Veggies, Spinach and Melty Cheese Sauce**

Prep Time: 15 mins
Cook Time: 20 mins

Ingredients: 1-pound boneless skinless chicken breasts or turkey breast (thinly sliced and pounded), 1/2 cup Greek yogurt, 8 ounces cheddar cheese (shredded), 1 teaspoon freshly squeezed lemon juice. 4 cups spinach, 1 tablespoon olive oil, 1/2 teaspoon sea salt, 1/2 teaspoon black pepper.

Preparation:
-Heat grill over medium heat, then lightly oil cooking grate. Grill chicken for about 10 minutes or until cooked through, then set aside on a plate.
-In a small mixing bowl combine Greek yogurt, cheese and lemon juice then microwave for about 30 seconds or until cheese is melted.
-In a large skillet, heat olive oil over medium heat, add spinach, and cook until wilted (about 2 minutes). Season with sea salt and black pepper if desired.
-To serve place chicken slices onto a plate, then top with spinach mixture and sauce.
-Enjoy!

DINNER: **Strawberry Shortcake**

Prep Time: 10 mins
Cook Time: 20 mins

Ingredients: 1 cup whole milk, 1/4 cup sugar, 1 package white cake mix, 4 cups frozen strawberries, 1 cup cool whip.

Preparation:
-Preheat oven to 375 degrees. In a medium bowl combine milk and sugar then add in cake mix and stir until well blended. Pour into a 10-inch round baking dish then bake in preheated oven for 20 minutes or until center is set. Remove from oven and set aside to cool completely. With an electric mixer beat on low-speed frozen strawberries until pureed and smooth then fold in cool whip.
-Using the same electric mixer beat on medium until layers of cake are fluffy and light (about 2 minutes). Spread strawberry filling over cake and on top then refrigerate until ready to serve.
-Enjoy!

DAY 29

BREAKFAST: **Taco Salad**

Prep Time: 10 mins
Cook Time: 1 hour

Ingredients: 4 cups kale or spinach (chopped), 1 1/2 cup cooked quinoa (warm), 8 ounces diced tomatoes (diced), 2 red onions (diced), 8 ounces cooked Italian sausage, 12 eggs. 2 jalapeno peppers (minced).

Preparation:

-Wash and trim kale or spinach to remove tough stems, then place into a large bowl. Add in quinoa and mix until coated then set aside. Heat a large skillet over high heat, then add in oil and heat until hot but not smoking. Add in sausage and cook for about 8 minutes or until browned, then set aside.
-Heat a large nonstick pan over medium-high heat then add in diced onions, jalapenos and tomatoes then cook for about 5 minutes or until softened. In a bowl whisk egg then pour into skillet. Cook for about 2 minutes without stirring or scramble should be firm but cooked through.
-To serve, place cooked quinoa and sausage on a large platter along with kale/spinach mixture, eggs, tomatoes, and onions.
-Enjoy!

LUNCH: **Italian Sausage and Tomato Scramble over Kale or Spinach**

Prep Time: 5 mins
Cook Time: 20 mins

Ingredients:3 tablespoons olive oil, 4 Italian sausages (sliced), 1/4 cup diced onion, 1/4 cup diced red bell pepper. 1 tablespoon minced garlic, 8 ounces cherry tomatoes (halved), 2 large eggs. 4 cups chopped kale or spinach, salt and pepper to taste.

Preparation:

-In a small skillet add in olive oil then sauté sausage until slightly browned, then set aside on a plate. Whisk eggs in a bowl, season with salt and pepper, and set aside.
-In a large heated skillet heat olive oil over medium heat and sauté onion, red bell pepper, and garlic until tender (about 7 minutes). Add in tomatoes and cook for about 10 minutes or until slightly softened.
-Remove from heat then add in eggs and scramble until cooked through. Add in sausage and stir to combine then serve immediately over kale or spinach.
-Enjoy!

DINNER: Strawberry Shortcake Muffins

Prep Time: 20 mins
Cook Time: 30 mins

Ingredients: 1 large white or yellow onion (chopped), 2 tablespoons olive oil, 2 pounds ground turkey breast (ground), 2 teaspoons salt, 2 teaspoons black pepper. 4 cups fresh strawberries (cut in half), 8 ounces low-fat cream cheese (softened). 1 package white cake mix, 2 tablespoons cornstarch. 1/4 cup water. 1/3 cup evaporated skim milk.

Preparation:
-Preheat oven to 350 degrees. Lightly grease a 12-count muffin tin or line with muffin liners, then set aside. -In a large bowl add in chopped onion, ground turkey and season with salt and pepper then combine using hands. -Line each muffin cup with cornstarch, use a spoon to fill each cup with turkey mixture, then place into the refrigerator while you prepare the strawberry topping.
-In a blender, puree strawberries with 1/4 cup water until smooth then set aside.
-In a large mixing bowl combine flour, cake mix, cornstarch and cream cheese until just combined. Add in strawberry sauce in small batches until combined and spreadable. If needed, place pan back on heat for about 15 seconds to warm slightly before pouring into muffin tin. Fill each tin about 3/4 of the way full. -Bake for about 25 minutes or until toothpick comes out clean. Cool for about 5 minutes then serve warm.

DAY 30

BREAKFAST: Fruit Pizza

Prep Time: 10 mins
Cook Time: 20 mins

Ingredients: 2 large eggs (beaten), 2 tablespoons milk, 1 teaspoon vanilla extract, 1 box pizza dough mix, 3/4 cup of fruit of choice.

Preparation:
-Heat oven to 375 degrees. Mix together eggs and milk then set aside. On a floured surface, roll out pizza dough into desired size, then use a sharp knife or pizza cutter to cut into desired size circles. Place on parchment paper lined cookie sheet then bake in preheated oven for about 8 minutes or until lightly browned. Remove from oven and set aside to cool.

-When dough is cooled spread egg mixture over pizza dough, then top with fruit that has been chopped into desired size. Serve warm or at room temperature.
-Enjoy!

LUNCH: **Spicy Chicken & Mushroom Wafflewich**

Prep Time: 15 mins
Cook Time: 10 mins

Ingredients: 1/2 cup chopped Bok choy, 1/4 cup thinly sliced mushrooms (I used baby Portobello), 3 tablespoons olive oil, 3 tablespoons ghee or butter, 2 garlic cloves (minced), 1 pound ground chicken, 2 teaspoons minced ginger. 1 teaspoon chili powder, 1/2 teaspoon salt. 2 eggs (beaten). 1/3 cup chopped cilantro. 1 tablespoon soy sauce (optional). 1 teaspoon sesame oil.

Preparation:

-Heat a large skillet over medium heat, then add in olive oil or ghee and garlic then sauté until fragrant. Add in mushrooms, then sauté for about 4 minutes or until soft and tender. In a small bowl combine eggs and soy sauce (if using) then set aside.
-Drain fat from spinach, then squeeze out any excess water into a small bowl. Chop spinach into bite sized pieces then set aside. Combine ground chicken with garlic, ginger, chili powder and salt then set aside. -In a large skillet, add spinach, eggs and chicken mixture, then cook for about 1 minute or until the egg is completely cooked through.
-Cut each waffle into 6 triangles and serve with bok choy and mushrooms in the center.
-Enjoy!

DINNER: **Strawberry Cream Cheese Cupcakes with Fresh Strawberries**

Prep Time: 15 mins
Cook Time: 25 mins

Ingredients: 1/2 cup low-fat cream cheese (softened), 1/4 cup granulated sugar, 1 egg yolk, 1 tablespoon milk, 2 teaspoons vanilla extract. 1 package white cake mix. A pinch of salt. 2 cups fresh strawberries (chopped), 2 teaspoons vanilla extract.

Preparation:

-Combine cream cheese and granulated sugar until completely combined then set aside. Whisk together egg yolk and milk, then set aside. -In a large bowl, combine flour, salt, cake mix, and vanilla, then stir until just combined. Add in egg mixture and mix until just combined; then add in chopped strawberries and fresh strawberries. -Divide into cupcake liners about 1/4 of the way full, then bake for about 25 minutes or until toothpick comes out clean. -Cool for about 5 minutes then serve warm.
-Enjoy!

DAY 31

BREAKFAST: Chicken Teriyaki with Rice and Broccoli

Prep Time: 15 mins
Cook Time: 40 mins

Ingredients: 1/4 cup low-sodium soy sauce, 2 tablespoons mirin (optional), 2 tablespoons honey, 2 teaspoons cornstarch, 1 clove garlic (minced), 3 boneless chicken breasts (thinly sliced or diced), 1 teaspoon salt, 1/4 teaspoon black pepper. 1 tablespoon sesame oil. 3 cups fresh broccoli florets. Steamed brown rice (cooked).

Preparation:
-In a bowl, combine soy sauce, mirin, and honey, mix until well combined, then set aside.
-In a small bowl combine dry ingredients then set aside. Add sesame oil and garlic in a large skillet, then sauté for about 1 minute or until fragrant. Add in chicken and mix with spoon to coat thoroughly without any burning. Cook over medium-high heat for about 3 minutes or until chicken is fully cooked through.
-Add steamed broccoli to skillet then cover with soy sauce mixture and cook for about 3 minutes or until chicken is fully cooked through.
-Place rice into bowls then top with teriyaki chicken and broccoli. Serve warm.
-Enjoy!

LUNCH: Strawberry Spinach Salad with Creamy Dill Dressing, Fresh Berries

Prep Time: 15 mins
Cook Time: 10 mins

Ingredients: 1 (16oz) package baby spinach, fresh strawberries (sliced), 3 tablespoons olive oil, 2 teaspoons fresh lemon juice. 2 tablespoons breadcrumbs. 1/3 cup chopped cilantro, 1 tablespoon shallot (minced), 2 teaspoons sugar. salt & pepper to taste, 1/2 cup reduced-fat plain Greek yogurt, 2 teaspoons minced garlic, 1/4 teaspoon black pepper, 1/2 teaspoon lemon pepper, 1/4 cup finely chopped fennel (optional).

Preparation:
Combine all ingredients in a salad bowl, then toss to coat. Serve immediately.
-Enjoy!

DINNER: Lemon Curd and Butter Shortbread Cookies

Prep Time: 10 mins
Cook Time: 30 mins

Ingredients: 1 stick butter at room temp, 3/4 cup sugar (granulated), 2 tablespoons fresh lemon juice, 2 large egg whites, 1 1/2 cups flour (all-purpose). A pinch of salt, 1 package Miss Meringue Pie Filling (lemon curd), and Fresh Berries for garnish.

Preparation:

-In a saucepan, add lemon juice and butter, over medium heat, then stir occasionally until butter is melted. In a bowl beat egg whites until stiff peaks form (about 5 minutes). Slowly add sugar and continue beating until desired stiff peaks form. In another bowl combine flour, salt, Miss Meringue Pie Filling and shortbread cookie dough. On a surface with floured hands (or parchment paper), combine the two by folding in 1/2 of the flour mixture until dough becomes smooth.
-Place dough into a pastry bag, then pipe dough onto parchment paper. Bake at 350 degrees Fahrenheit for about 20 -25 minutes or until golden brown. Let cool for 5 minutes and serve with fresh fruit.
-Enjoy!

DAY 32

BREAKFAST: Beef Stir-fry with Snow Peas and Mushrooms

Prep Time: 15 mins
Cook Time: 20 mins

Ingredients: 1 medium onion (chopped), 5-6 ounces thinly sliced beef sirloin, 8 ounces white mushrooms, 1 teaspoon olive oil. 1 medium carrot (sliced), 2 cups fresh snow peas (snap peas), 2 teaspoons minced garlic, A pinch of salt. 1/4 cup low-sodium soy sauce (optional), 2 tablespoons corn starch mixed with a dash of water.
-In a large skillet over medium-high heat, add in olive oil, garlic and onions, then sauté for about 3 minutes or until fragrant. Add beef, carrots, and mushrooms, then cook for about 2 minutes. Stir frequently to avoid burning.
-Add tomato paste, soy sauce and corn starch mixture, then stir well to combine. Cook for about 5 minutes or until mixture becomes thickened slightly.
-Add snow peas to skillet then cook for another 2 minutes or until vegetables are tender yet crisp. Serve warm while hot.
-Enjoy!

LUNCH: **Baked Eggs with Avocado & Tomato**

Prep Time: 10 mins
Cook Time: 20 mins

Ingredients: 4 cups (12 oz) diced tomatoes or 1 can (14.5 oz) diced tomatoes, 1/2 tablespoon fresh basil, 2 cloves garlic (minced), salt and pepper to taste, 2 teaspoons extra-virgin olive oil, 4 large eggs, 1/4 cup grated cheese of choice, 2 tablespoons chopped parsley.

Preparation:
-Preheat oven to 400 degrees F, then line a baking sheet with aluminum foil and set aside.
-In a large bowl combine tomatoes and basil then set aside. In another large bowl beat eggs. Add salt, pepper and garlic then mix well.
-Pour egg mixture into the baking dish, then place the tomatoes into the dish and sprinkle cheese on top. Bake for about 15 -20 minutes or until the eggs are firm but still moist on top.
-In a small skillet, warm up tomato mixture over medium heat, then serve warm with baked eggs and garnish with parsley if desired.
-Enjoy!

DINNER: **Paleo Pecan Pie**

Prep Time: 15 mins
Cook Time: 45 mins

Ingredients: For the crust 1/3 cup raw almonds (pounded in a food processor), 1/4 cup coconut flour, 1/2 teaspoon vanilla, pinch of salt. For the filling 6 eggs (separated), 2 tablespoons ghee or coconut oil for topping, 1 tablespoon chocolate chips and toffee bits.

Preparation:
-Preheat oven to 325 degrees F then line a 9 inch pie pan with aluminum foil and set aside.
-In a large food processor, combine almonds and coconut flour then mash until almonds are lightly ground. Add in vanilla and salt and continue to pulse until dough is well combined.
-Spoon dough into the prepared pie pan then bake for about 15 -20 minutes or until the center of pie rises a bit (about 6 inches). In a medium bowl, cream sugar with vanilla and eggs until light, then mix chocolate chips and toffee bits.
-Remove pie from oven then pour filling into the crust before returning it to the oven for another 5 minutes or until filling is set (whipped peaks will be formed). Remove pie from oven then sprinkle the ghee on top before serving while still warm.
-Enjoy!

DAY 33

BREAKFAST: **Grilled Salmon with Asparagus and Quinoa**

Prep Time: 15 mins
Cook Time: 20 mins

Ingredients: 1-2 lbs. salmon filet, For the sauce 2 teaspoons olive oil, 1 shallot (minced), 2 cloves of garlic (minced), 2 tablespoons grain free chicken broth, salt and pepper to taste. For the vegetables 3 cups asparagus (cut into 1-inch pieces), 5 ounces of mushrooms, 1 cup quinoa or white rice.

Preparation:
-Preheat oven 400 degrees F, then mix all ingredients for the sauce in a bowl. -Season salmon with salt and pepper. -Toss veggies in olive oil until coated, then place on a baking sheet. Bake for about 15 - 20 minutes or until tender. -In a large skillet over medium heat, add in oil and shallot. Fry for about 1 -2 minutes then add in garlic, grain free chicken broth, salt and pepper.
-Once broth begins to boil, reduce heat to low and let simmer (keep lid on) while cooking the fish.
-Once the sauce becomes thickened add quinoa to the pan then stir well to combine. Cook for another 3 - 5 minutes or until quinoa is tender yet firm to bite.
-Remove fish from oven, then top with the asparagus, quinoa and mushrooms. Cook for another 2 minutes or until fish is cooked to perfection.
-Serve warm with a fork and knife.
-Enjoy!

LUNCH: **Quiche Lorraine (Paleo)**

Prep Time: 10 mins
Cook Time: 45 mins

Ingredients: 8 ounces lean ground beef, 1 tablespoon Paleo mayo, 1 cup of low carb tomato sauce, 6 large eggs. 1/2 cup shredded cheese of choice (I recommend mozzarella).

Preparation:
Preheat oven to 350 degrees F, spray a 9-inch pie dish with olive oil, and set aside.
-In a medium bowl combine the ground beef, Paleo mayo, diced tomatoes and seasonings for the sauce. Mix well until well combined.
-In a separate bowl, cream eggs with remaining ingredients, then add in beef mixture then stir till well combined. -Pour into prepared dish and bake for about 30 -35 minutes or until set (center will still jiggle a bit). Serve while hot with a fork and knife.
-Enjoy!

DINNER: **Paleo Apple Crisp (Paleo)**

Prep Time: 1 hour
Cook Time: 20 mins

Ingredients: 4 large apples (Peel, core, and slice into about 1/4-inch-thick slices), 2 tablespoons ghee or coconut oil, 2 tablespoons coconut sugar or pure maple syrup. 1 teaspoon cinnamon. 1/4 cup ground almonds

Preparation:

-Preheat the oven to 350 degrees F, then grease a 9 x 13 baking dish with olive oil and set aside.
-In a medium bowl, combine all ingredients then pour evenly into the baking dish.
-Bake for about 20 -25 minutes or until apples are tender yet crisp. -Serve warm with a fork and knife.
-Enjoy!

DAY 34

BREAKFAST: **Lemon Garlic Chicken with Roasted potatoes and green beans**

Prep Time: 10 mins
Cook Time: 40 mins

Ingredients: 3 large or 4 small chicken breasts (thawed, skinned, seasoned with salt, pepper, garlic powder, onion powder), 2 tablespoons ghee or coconut oil, 1/2 medium sweet potato (sliced into thin rounds), 1/2 small zucchini (sliced into thin rounds), 2 cups fresh spinach leaves. 1 cup fresh cranberries. 2 tablespoons fresh basil. 1 cup mushrooms, 1/2 cup bell peppers (small thin slices), 1/2 cup fresh basil leaves, 1 teaspoon oregano, 1/8 teaspoon black pepper.

Preparation:

-In a large skillet over medium heat, heat the ghee or coconut oil.
-Once heated add in seasoned chicken breasts then cook for about 8 -10 minutes on each side or until cooked through (175 degrees F internal temp). -Remove chicken from skillet then allow to rest on a plate. -In the same skillet over the same medium heat, add in sliced zucchini and sweet potatoes then cook for about 5 -8 minutes or until tender.
-Remove from heat then top with fried chicken breasts.
-In a large bowl, toss together the spinach, cranberries, basil, mushrooms, bell peppers and basil leaves. Season with oregano and black pepper then top with chicken for serving.
-Enjoy!

LUNCH: **Pepperoni Pizza Pita Sandwich with Oregano Tomato Salad**

Prep Time: 10 mins
Cook Time: 25 mins

Ingredients: 1/3 cup olive oil or avocado oil, 1 tablespoon red wine vinegar, 1 lemon (juice only), 2 tablespoons chopped sun-dried tomatoes (optional), salt and pepper to taste, 1 large tomato (cored and chopped into small chunks), 3 -4 large romaine lettuce hearts, pepperoni sticks, oregano for topping, 1 red bell pepper (roasted, peeled and sliced).

Preparation:
-In a small bowl, combine oil, vinegar, lemon juice, and sun-dried tomatoes. Season with salt and pepper as desired then set aside.
-In a large bowl toss together the tomatoes and lettuce. Top with dressing then add pepperoni sticks and roasted red bell peppers.
-Sprinkle with oregano and enjoy.
-Enjoy!

DINNER: **Chocolate Caramel Brownies with Coconut Flakes & Dark Chocolate Chips**

Prep Time: 20 mins
Cook Time: 60 mins

Ingredients: 1/2 cup coconut flour, 1/4 cup arrowroot flour or tapioca starch, 1 teaspoon baking powder, 2 teaspoons vanilla extract, 1 3/4 cups dark chocolate chips or 3 ounces of 70 percent cacao chocolate bar. 1/2 cup chopped walnuts. 1/2 cup coconut palm sugar or pure maple syrup, 3 eggs. 1/2 cup unsweetened baking cocoa powder or unsweetened cocoa powder (to make raw), 1 tablespoon pure vanilla extract, 1 tablespoon apple cider vinegar, 2 teaspoons flax oil or ground flax seeds.

Preparation:
-Preheat oven to 350 degrees F, then grease a 9 x 13 baking dish with olive oil and set aside.
-In a large bowl combine all ingredients with the exception of flax oil or ground flax seeds and mix well until well combined and smooth then add in flax oil and mix again till combined.
-Pour batter into baking dish and bake for about 35 -40 minutes or until center is no longer jiggly. (I prefer my brownies a little chewy so I took it out of the oven at 35 minutes, but if you like yours more done then leave in oven for up to 40 minutes).
-Remove from oven and allow to cool for 10 -15 minutes before cutting into squares. Enjoy with a fork and knife.
-Enjoy!

DAY 35

BREAKFAST: **Pesto Chicken Salad Wrap with roasted peppers, mozzarella cheese, and arugula leaves**

Prep Time: 10 mins
Cook Time: 10 mins

Ingredients: 1/4 cup olive oil or avocado oil, 1 tablespoon red wine vinegar, 2 tablespoons chopped sun-dried tomatoes (optional), salt and pepper to taste, 1 large tomato (cored and chopped into small chunks), 2 -3 large romaine lettuce hearts. 1/2 cup fresh basil leaves. 6-7 sliced chicken breasts (cooked by choice). Pepperoni sticks or bacon pieces for topping. Mozzarella cheese slices for topping.

Preparation:

-In a small bowl, combine oil, vinegar, lemon juice, and sun-dried tomatoes. Season with salt and pepper as desired then set aside. -In a large bowl, toss together the lettuce and tomatoes, then add chicken breasts and basil leaves. Top with dressing then add pepperoni sticks, bacon slices or mozzarella cheese slices for serving.

LUNCH: **Veggie Frittata with Egg & Tomato**

Prep Time: 10 mins
Cook Time: 15 mins

Ingredients: 1/2 medium zucchini (sliced into thin rounds), 1/2 medium sweet potato (cut into thin rounds), 1/2 cup mushrooms, 2 cups fresh spinach leaves, 2 large eggs. 1/4 cup olive oil or avocado oil, 2 tablespoons red wine vinegar, salt and pepper to taste. 3 medium tomatoes (cored and chopped into small chunks). 4 slices of bacon (crumbled). 4 ounces mozzarella cheese (shredded). 1/4 cup fresh basil leaves, oregano for topping.

Preparation:

-In a large skillet over medium heat, add oil, vinegar and sun-dried tomatoes. Season with salt and pepper as desired, then add zucchini, sweet potatoes, mushrooms, and spinach leaves. Cook until tender (about 6 -10 minutes). Remove from heat then top with fried chicken breasts. Preheat the broiler on your oven then set the oven rack to the highest position (about 6 inches below the heat source). -In a medium bowl whisk together eggs and season with salt and pepper as desired. -In a

small baking dish (I used a 10 x 7 rectangular dish), spread out the chopped tomatoes then top with crumbled bacon. -Evenly pour egg mixture over bacon then add shredded mozzarella cheese on top. -Place baking dish into the oven and broil for about 2 -3 minutes or until top is lightly browned. -Remove from oven and allow to cool before cutting into squares. Top with fresh basil leaves and oregano for serving.
Enjoy!

DINNER: **Paleo Pumpkin Tart**
Prep Time: 10 mins
Cook Time: 40 mins

Ingredients: 1 cup almond flour or blanched almond flour (or you can use 2/3 cup coconut flour), 3 tablespoons pure maple syrup, 1 teaspoon ground cinnamon, 1/4 teaspoon grated nutmeg, salt to taste, 3 large eggs. 1/4 cup olive oil or avocado oil, 2 tablespoons red wine vinegar. 1 medium pie pumpkin (cored and chopped into small chunks). 4 ounces mozzarella cheese (shredded). 4 slices of bacon (crumbled). Pre-cooked sausage links for topping.

Preparation:
-Preheat oven to 325 degrees F, then grease a 10 x 15 baking dish with olive oil and set aside.
-In a large bowl, combine almond flour or blanched almond flour, cinnamon, nutmeg, salt and eggs; beat with an electric mixer until smooth. Slowly add oil (or avocado oil) and vinegar then continue to beat until well combined. -Spread batter into the prepared baking dish and about 1/4 cup at a time into the dish (spacing out the batter). Top with pumpkin chunks and mozzarella cheese then sprinkle with crumbled bacon. -Bake for about 40 - 45 minutes or until center is no longer jiggly.
-Remove from oven and allow to cool for 10 -15 minutes before cutting into squares.
-Enjoy!

DAY 36

BREAKFAST: **Cobb Salad with grilled chicken, bacon, hard-boiled eggs, avocado, blue cheese, and tomato**
Prep Time: 10 mins
Cook Time: 5 mins

Ingredients: 1/2 cup shredded brussels sprouts, 1 Roma tomato (diced), 2 -3 tablespoons fresh basil leaves (tear into small pieces), 3 -4 large romaine lettuce hearts (washed and dried with paper towels then divided between serving dishes). 6 slices of cooked bacon (thinly sliced into pieces). 4 medium eggs (beaten in a large bowl until egg mixture is well mixed). 1/2 cup fresh parsley leaves. Salt & Pepper to taste. 1/4 cup olive oil or avocado oil, 2 tablespoons red wine vinegar, 1/2 cup crumbled blue cheese. 1/2 pound chicken breasts (cooked and cut into thin strips).

Preparation:

In a large bowl, whisk together egg mixture until well combined, then add salt and pepper as desired. In a separate small bowl, combine lemon juice and maple syrup, then set aside.
-In a large skillet over medium heat, add oil, vinegar and sun-dried tomatoes. Season with salt and pepper as desired then add brussels sprouts. Cook until tender (about 3 -5 minutes). Remove from heat then top with cooked chicken slices. -In a medium bowl, mix blue cheese and maple syrup, then add basil, tomato and parsley. Stir well then divide between serving dishes.
-Place 2 slices of bacon into each serving dish. Top with egg mixture then sprinkle with crumbled blue cheese for serving.
Enjoy!

LUNCH: **French Toast Sticks with Syrup and Bananas**
Prep Time: 15 mins
Cook Time: 5 mins

Ingredients: 1 cup coconut flour or almond flour, 1 teaspoon baking powder, 1/4 teaspoon sea salt, 2 large eggs (beaten in a small bowl until well mixed). 3 tablespoons coconut oil or pure olive oil, 2 tablespoons apple cider vinegar or lemon juice (to taste). 1 cup fresh pineapple (sliced into thin strips). 3 large eggs (beaten with a fork). 1/4 cup honey or pure maple syrup.

Preparation:
-In a medium bowl, whisk together flour, baking powder and sea salt. Set aside.
-In a large bowl, cream together oil and vinegar until well combined then add pineapple and eggs. Beat until mixture is well mixed, then stir in honey or maple syrup until well combined.
-Heat the skillet over medium-high heat, then add coconut or olive oil. Place a large spoonful of batter into the skillet for each piece of chicken breast (about 2 -3 tablespoons per piece). Spread batter out over the oiled skillet then cook until golden brown (about 3-5 minutes per side).
-Remove from heat and allow to cool. Serve with cut up pineapple, maple syrup and honey for dipping.

DINNER: **Paleo Lemon Meringue Pie**
Prep Time: 15 mins
Cook Time: 5 mins

Ingredients: 1/2 cup unsalted butter, 8-ounce package cream cheese, 2 large egg yolks. 2 teaspoons lemon zest (zest from 1 lemon). 1 teaspoon pure vanilla extract. 1/4 cup fresh lemon juice. 2/3 cup fresh blueberries (you can use frozen berries as well). 3 large egg whites with a pinch of cream of tartar. 1/2 cup honey (or pure maple syrup)

Preparation:

-In a small bowl, beat together butter and cream cheese until well combined. Add vanilla extract and lemon zest, then beat until smooth. Set aside.

-In another medium sized bowl, beat egg yolks with a hand blender until well blended then add honey or maple syrup and continue to mix until well blended. Add lemon juice and combine thoroughly then set aside. -In the same bowl, beat egg whites with a hand blender until well mixed then add cream of tartar and mix on high speed for about 30 seconds to make stiff peaks (will take about 1 hour to achieve stiff peaks). -Now make sure your oven is preheated to 350 degrees F.

-Now transfer half the batter into a piping bag fitted with an open star tip. Pipe whipped cream into the prepared spring form pan into 1" mounds.

-Add blueberries to the remaining batter and blend until well combined then transfer into another piping bag. Pipe dollops of whipped cream on top of the lemon meringue pie and garnish with blueberries. Drizzle honey or maple syrup for serving.

-Place spring form pan into a deep baking dish, then place in the oven to bake for about 5 minutes. Place the pie onto a cake plate and serve immediately with honey or maple syrup.

-Enjoy!

DAY 37

BREAKFAST: **Turkey stuffing balls with cranberry sauce**

Prep Time: 10 mins
Cook Time: 45 mins

Ingredients: 1 1/2 lbs. ground turkey (80% lean), 1/2 cup chopped celery 1/8 cup chopped scallions (green onions) 2 tsp dried rosemary 2 tbsp. fresh parsley, chopped 2 tbsp. fresh sage, chopped 6 slices bacon (cooked and crumbled into small pieces). 1/3 cup olive oil salt and pepper to taste. 6 large eggs (beaten in a large bowl). 1/2 cup almond flour (or coconut flour).

Preparation:

-In a large bowl, combine turkey, celery, and scallions, then gently mix with a spoon. Add sage and parsley, then gently mix (do not overmix). Season with salt & pepper as desired.

-Lay out 6 pieces of bacon on paper towel to dry out excess grease. Preheat oven to 425 degrees F and cook the bacon until crispy. Set aside.
-In a medium sized bowl, whisk together eggs with salt & pepper then add rosemary, sage, celery and scallions' mixture evenly among eggs (no need to completely mix everything).
-Transfer eggs into a greased 10" pie pan then sprinkle with crumbled bacon.
-Bake in the oven for 20-25 minutes, then serve with your favorite sauce (citrus orange marmalade/ fresh cranberry sauce). Enjoy!

LUNCH: **Frittata with Bacon, Spinach, Turkey and Melted Cheese**

Prep Time: 15 mins
Cook Time: 25 mins

Ingredients: 4 large eggs, 2 tbsp ghee 2 oz cheese (your choice) 1 cup chopped spinach (you can use frozen spinach as well), 3 slices bacon (cooked and crumbled into small pieces), 1/2 cup tomato sauce, salt and pepper to taste, 1 tsp dried basil, 1/4 tsp dried oregano.

Preparation:
-Preheat oven to 375 degrees F.
-In a medium sized bowl, add eggs and beat thoroughly with a fork to mix.
-Add ghee into the bowl then add spinach evenly over the top of eggs. Mix until blended well.
-Transfer egg mixture into a greased 10" pie pan then sprinkle with crumbled bacon.
-Bake in the oven for 12 - 15 minutes, then remove from oven and top with cheese and tomato sauce. Sprinkle dried basil and oregano over the top of frittata and serve immediately. Enjoy!

DINNER: **Paleo Peach Tart**

Prep Time: 10 mins
Cook Time: 35 mins

Ingredients: 1 pie crust (your choice). 1/2 cup butter (melted), 1 9" unbaked pie shell, 3 cups fresh peaches (cut into small pieces), 1/4 cup lemon juice, 2 cups chopped almonds (chopped - but not too fine), pinch of sea salt, pinch of ground nutmeg, pinch of cinnamon.

Preparation:
-Prepare pie crust and preheat greased pie dish by placing a piece of parchment paper over the bottom of the dish and placing a piece of foil on top to prevent the bottom from getting burned then place on the middle rack in your preheated oven.
-In a medium sized bowl, add melted butter, chopped peaches and lemon juice then mix well.
-Place the pie shell in the preheated oven then add peach mixture into the preheated pie shell.
-Bake on the middle rack in your oven for 20 - 25 minutes until crust is lightly golden brown on top.
-Sprinkle with chopped almonds, sea salt, nutmeg and cinnamon to taste then serve with a slice of fresh ripe peach for dipping. Enjoy!

DAY 38

BREAKFAST: **Shepherd's Pie**

Prep Time: 20 mins
Cook Time: 10 mins

Ingredients: 3 large eggs + 3 large egg whites (beaten) 1 1/2 cups lean ground beef, 1/2 cup chopped bell peppers (red, green, yellow). 1/4 cup chopped onions, 2 tbsp olive oil (extra virgin), salt and pepper to taste, 1 cup tomato sauce, 2 large carrots (finely sliced), pinch of cayenne red pepper flakes, 2 tbsp fresh parsley, chopped, 2 tsp dried oregano powder, 1 tsp dried dill weed (or two sprigs fresh dill weed if you have it).

Preparation:

-In a large bowl, add beef, bell peppers, onions and olive oil. Season with salt & pepper as desired. Gently mix with a spoon until well combined (no need to completely mix everything).
-In a medium sized bowl, beat eggs and egg whites with a fork, then add meat mixture and make sure it is evenly distributed among the eggs & whites. Make sure there are no egg yolks in the bottom of the bowl.
-Add chopped carrots, tomato sauce, and all other seasonings together into one bowl, then mix through (do not overmix).
-Line a baking dish with parchment paper. In the baking dish, add meat mixture then top with carrot mixture. Bake in the oven for 15 - 20 mins at 350 degrees F until carrots are soft and tender and golden brown. -Remove from oven, add fresh parsley flakes and serve. Enjoy!

LUNCH: **Southwest Quiche**

Prep Time: 10 mins
Cook Time: 25 mins

Ingredients: 2 large eggs + 2 large egg whites (beaten with fork) 3/4 cup cooked chicken (finely chopped) 1 cup chopped bell pepper (red, green, yellow), 1/4 cup chopped onions, 4 fresh slices of jalapeño pepper, 1/4 tsp each of sea salt and black pepper, 1/8 tsp cayenne red pepper flakes (if you want a spicy quiche, omit the red pepper flakes), 1 1/2 cups grated low-fat mozzarella (or your favorite cheese), salt and pepper to taste, 1/4 cup sliced green onions.

Preparation:

-Preheat oven to 350 degrees F, then prepare your pie crust and preheat the oven to 350 degrees F as well. In a large bowl, add eggs, egg whites, chicken, bell peppers, onions and sea salt & pepper as desired then gently stir together with a fork until just mixed (no need to completely mix everything).
-In a separate large bowl, add mozzarella cheese, cayenne red pepper flakes (if you want a spicy quiche), salt & pepper as desired.
-Spread the quiche mixture into your prepared pie crust then sprinkle with cheese and sliced green onions. Bake in oven for 25 - 30 mins until the edges of the quiche are browned and the cheese is melted. Let cool and serve. Enjoy!

DINNER: Chocolate Almond Cupcakes with Coconut Flakes & Dark Chocolate Chips with Fresh Strawberries

Prep Time: 10 mins
Cook Time: 30 mins

Ingredients: 2 cups blanched almond flour (finely ground) 2 tsp baking soda 1/4 tsp sea salt (or Himalayan pink rock salt), 1/4 cup raw honey or your favorite sweetener for paleo, 1/4 cup melted butter (or ghee for Paleo), 4 large whole eggs, 2 large egg whites, 1/2 tsp vanilla extract, 3 tbsp almond butter, 3 tbsp coconut oil (melted) 1/2 cup dark chocolate chips, 6 fresh strawberries (chopped).

Preparation:
-In a medium sized bowl, add the almond flour, baking soda and sea salt then mix through.
-In a large bowl, mix the honey and melted butter, add almond butter, and mix again.
-Add eggs and egg whites to the large bowl, then mix all ingredients together until well combined.
-Add wet ingredients into dry ingredients then mix thoroughly, preferably with an electric mixer (this will ensure no lumps).
-Preheat oven to 350 degrees F and prepare your cupcake pan by lining each cup with parchment paper (do not grease the pan).
-Pour batter evenly into each cupcake mold until 2/3 full. Give batter a few taps on the counter to remove any air bubbles and smooth out.
-Place the cupcake pan on the middle rack in your preheated oven.
-Bake for 15 - 20 minutes until a tooth pick comes out clean. Remove from oven and let cool in the cupcake pan then place in refrigerator until ready to serve.
-Before serving, top each cupcake with melted chocolate chips, chopped strawberries and coconut flakes for garnish (optional). Enjoy!

DAY 39

BREAKFAST: Chicken Pot Pie

Prep Time: 15 mins
Cook Time: 35 mins

Ingredients: 1 large egg + 1 large egg white (beaten) 1/4 cup chopped green onions, 1 cup sliced carrots (matchsticks), 1/4 cup chopped button mushrooms, 3 tbsp coconut oil, 2 cups finely shredded, cooked chicken (or salmon), salt and pepper to taste, water for boiling the vegetables.

Preparation:

-In a large bowl, add eggs and egg whites with a fork, then season with salt & pepper as desired.
-Heat a pot of boiling water until it is hot (do not add sea salt). In the pot, place sliced carrots and green onions then remove once they become soft (approx. 3 mins). Place back into the egg mixture with mushrooms and chicken (or salmon) then set aside.
-In a separate pot, heat coconut oil on medium high heat until melted (do not add sea salt).
-Gently pour egg mixture into a pot of coconut oil and cook until it solidifies around the edges (approx. 1 minute). Once solid, flip over and cook the other side. Remove from oil with a spatula then place in your serving bowl. Repeat steps 4 - 6 with remaining egg mixture.
-Preheat oven to 400 degrees F and line a baking dish (pie dish or cake pan) with parchment paper.
-In your serving bowl, add the cooked egg mixture and sprinkle with salt & pepper. Bake in the oven for 5 - 10 minutes until the top of the egg mixture is golden brown.
-Top with fresh parsley flakes and serve. Enjoy!

LUNCH: Shrimp Scampi in Pita Bread or Lettuce Wrap with Cucumber and Tomato Salad

Prep Time: 15 mins
Cook Time: 10 mins

Ingredients: 6 large shrimp, 1/2 tbsp coconut oil, 1/4 cup chopped red onions (finely chopped), 3 garlic cloves (minced), 2 tsp capers, 1/2 tbsp dried oregano, 1 tsp lemon juice, freshly ground sea salt & pepper to taste.

Preparation:

-In a large pan on medium heat, add olive oil and cook shrimp for 2-3 mins (do not overcook the shrimp or it will be tough). -In a small bowl, mix olive oil, red onions, garlic cloves and capers, then gently heat on medium-low until onions are soft (approx 3 mins). Add oregano. Squeeze lemon juice over top and season with sea salt & pepper as desired.

Prepare your pita bread or lettuce wrap by filling with 1 - 2 pieces of shrimp, cucumber and tomato slices, then drizzle with lemon juice and olive oil for garnish. Enjoy!

DINNER: Gingerbread Cookies (vegan, low carb)

Prep Time: 15 mins
Cook Time: 20 mins

Ingredients: 2 tbsp coconut oil, 1/3 cup almond butter, 1/3 cup cocoa powder, 1 large egg (well beaten), 1 tsp vanilla extract, pinch of sea salt & baking soda.

Preparation:
-In a large bowl, add combined almond butter and cocoa powder, then whisk together with a fork. Stir in the rest of your ingredients and mix until smooth like cake batter. If the batter is too thick to spread out on parchment paper, add water 1 tbsp at a time to thin it out.
-Line a baking sheet (preferably parchment paper) with baking paper. Spoon out batter and use a small offset spatula to spread out/smooth into cookie shape. If the batter is too thick, you may need to add water to thin it out.
-Bake in the oven for 18 - 20 minutes until edges are browned. Cool down, remove from baking sheet, and place on a serving plate for garnish.
-Top with chopped pecans and drizzle with chocolate, if desired. Enjoy!

DAY 40

BREAKFAST: Loaded Baked Potato Soup

Prep Time: 15 mins
Cook Time: 40 mins

Ingredients: 2 large russet potatoes, 2 cans of beans (such as black beans or kidney beans), 1 cup vegetable broth, 1/2 small onion (chopped), 1/2 cup corn kernels (fresh or frozen), 3 tbsp extra virgin olive oil, fresh parsley flakes, sea salt and fresh cracked pepper to taste.

Preparation:
-In a large pan over medium heat add olive oil and chopped onion then cook until soft and translucent (approx. 3 mins). Add potatoes to the pan and stir gently until they are cooked through. Season with salt & pepper as desired.

-Add vegetable broth to the pan, then add beans and corn, cover and cook for 3 - 5 mins (until potatoes break apart). Once the potato is cooked through, remove the lid and stir gently. Remove from heat.
-In a food processor box, add all ingredients, then process until smooth (approx. 20 seconds).
-Garnish with fresh parsley flakes and serve. Enjoy!

LUNCH: **Shrimp Stir-Fry with Brown Rice and Veggies**

Prep Time: 15 mins
Cook Time: 20 mins

Ingredients: 1 lb. raw shrimp, 1/2 tbsp olive oil, 1/4 cup onion (chopped), 1 head of broccoli (cut into florets), 2 cups cauliflower florets and 2 cups green beans (peeled and chopped).

Preparation:
-In a frying pan set over medium heat, drizzle olive oil then add onion then cook until soft (approx. 3 mins).
-Add broccoli and cauliflower, stir once cooked through.
-Add green beans and stir together.
-Season with sea salt & pepper to taste.
-Serve in bowls with brown rice. Enjoy!

DINNER: **Homemade Seitan Burgers & Chicken Fried Cauliflower Tots with Bacon Mac and Cheese (vegan & gluten free)**

Prep Time: 20 mins
Cook Time: 20 mins

Ingredients: 1/4 cup coconut oil, 1/4 cup almond flour, 3 cups vital wheat gluten, 2 cups hot water, 2 tbsp olive oil, 1/2 tsp oregano, 1/2 tsp paprika, salt and ground pepper to taste.

Preparation:
-In a large bowl, add coconut oil, almond flour and 3/4 cup of vital wheat gluten. Mix together with a fork then add oregano, paprika, salt and pepper.
-Add 1 cup of the hot water to the bowl, then use your hands to knead together until dough begins to form (approx. 10 mins). If dough is too dry or crumbly, add more water 1 tbsp at a time as needed.
-Once the dough is formed, cover bowl with a damp kitchen towel & allow it to rest for 15 minutes (this will help make your burger patties).
-In a pan over medium heat, add coconut oil and add in remaining 1/3 cup vital wheat gluten, then stir until combined (approx. 2 mins). Turn off heat then stir through the rest of the ingredients in the bowl with a spatula.

-Take approx. 1 tbsp of dough and roll into burger shape (do not over work the dough or it will become too hard to handle). Place on parchment paper. Repeat until all your dough has been used up. You may want to freeze any remaining dough for later use in other recipes such as scones, etc.

-Stir fry patties for approx. 5 mins per side or until browned.

-In a large skillet, add 1 tbsp of olive oil and add in cooked seitan patties.

-Fry for about 5 mins or until browned (do not overcook), then remove from skillet and set aside.

-In the same pan, add bacon bits and sauté for approx. 5 mins or until browned, then remove from pan.

-Then place cooked seitan patty with bacon bits on top of macaroni & cheese (top with more cheddar cheese if desired). Serve with extra bacon bits and parsley on the side to garnish.

DAY 41

BREAKFAST: Fried Rice with shrimp, chicken, and vegetables

Prep Time: 15 mins
Cook Time: 30 mins

Ingredients: 1 tbsp vinegar, 2 tablespoons soy sauce, 2 teaspoons vegetable oil, 1/4 cup green onions (several), 1 lb of cooked shrimp (peeled & diced), 8 ounces chicken breast (cooked and sliced), 8-ounce carrots (sliced into sticks) and 4 ounces sprouts (chop off ends).

Preparation:

-In a frying pan set over medium heat, add vegetable oil, then add onions & green onions. Season with sea salt and fresh cracked pepper to taste, then cook for about 5 mins or until tender. Turn off heat then set aside. -Add chicken, carrots, and sprouts to the same pan then season with soy sauce, vinegar and vegetable oil. Season with sea salt and fresh cracked pepper to taste.

-Turn heat back on at medium-high (approx. 5), then add shrimp. Stir for a few mins until cooked through then remove from heat. -To serve, plate rice, then top with shrimp, chicken, carrots & sprouts mixture. Garnish with green onion then serve. Enjoy!

LUNCH: Greek Chicken Pitas with Feta Cheese and Tzatziki Sauce

Prep Time: 10 mins
Cook Time: 30 mins

Ingredients: 2 cups cooked chicken breast, 2 bell peppers (red/yellow), 1 cup cucumber (sliced lengthwise), 1 cup cherry tomatoes, 3 tbsp extra virgin olive oil, Tzatziki Sauce, sea salt and pepper to taste.

Preparation:
-In a large bowl, add cucumber slices, then drizzle with 1 tbsp of olive oil, then season with sea salt and fresh cracked pepper to taste. Set aside.
-In a large pot of boiling water, add cherry tomatoes, then boil for 30 seconds. Remove and submerge into ice water for about 20 seconds or until it cools down. Snap off the ends of each tomato, then slice in half lengthwise (remove seeds). Set aside.
-In a large bowl, add 1/4 cup of olive oil, then squeeze of lemon juice, add crushed garlic and dill. Season with sea salt and fresh cracked pepper to taste. Mix well then set aside.
-Next, slice the bell peppers into strips then set aside.
-Add remaining ingredients in the order mentioned above (chicken breast > cucumbers > cherry tomatoes > bell peppers).
-Drizzle pita bread with 2 tbsp of olive oil, then toast in the oven for 3 mins (place it under broil until browned). Remove from oven and fill each pita pocket with chicken salad mixture & garnish with tomatoes and cucumber slices on top. Serve with tzatziki sauce on the side. Enjoy!

DINNER: Ground Lamb Vindaloo

Prep Time: 20 mins
Cook Time: 20 mins

Ingredients: 1 tbsp olive oil, 2 onions (sliced), 3 cloves garlic (minced), 1 red pepper (diced), 1 green pepper (diced), 2 cups tomato sauce, 4 tsp paprika, 4 tsp cayenne pepper (try a drop of chili oil for extra heat), 1/4 cup coconut milk, cooked seitan chunks, sea salt and pepper to taste.
Preparation:
-In a large pot, add oil then sauté onions, garlic and peppers until tender (approx 5 mins). Season with sea salt and fresh cracked pepper to taste. Set aside.
-In the same pot over medium heat, add paprika and cayenne pepper (to taste) then stir well. Add in tomato sauce, then bring to a boil.
-Once boiling, lower down heat to simmer for about 15 mins then add coconut milk. Season with sea salt and fresh cracked pepper to taste.
-Add cooked seitan chunks then simmer for 5 more mins or until all ingredients are heated through (seitan may need another 5 mins). Serve immediately with rice. Enjoy!

DAY 42

BREAKFAST: Spanish Vegetable Omelette

Prep Time: 15 mins
Cook Time: 20 mins

Ingredients: 3 tomatoes (diced), 2 onions (sliced), 1 red pepper (diced), 3 tbsp olive oil, 1 cup spinach (chopped), 8 eggs, sea salt and fresh cracked pepper to taste.

Preparation:
-In a large pot of boiling water, add tomatoes, then boil for 30 seconds. Remove and submerge into ice water for about 20 seconds or until it cools. Snap off the ends of each tomato, then slice in half lengthwise (remove seeds). Set aside.
-In a large bowl, add 2 tbsp olive oil and squeeze of lemon juice then whisk together well. Add onions, red pepper and season with sea salt and fresh cracked pepper to taste. Mix well then set aside.
-In the same bowl, add spinach, then season with sea salt and fresh cracked pepper to taste.
-In a medium pot (non-stick if possible), add eggs, then season with sea salt and fresh cracked pepper to taste. Add olive oil mixture and mix well. Remove from heat & set aside.
-In a large nonstick skillet, add tomato sauce then bring to a boil (lower heat). Once boiling, pour in egg mixture & cook for about 2 mins on each side or until well cooked.
-Split omelette evenly between 2 plates then top with spinach mixture on top. Serve immediately. Enjoy!

LUNCH: Creamy Lemon Chicken Wrap

Prep Time: 15 mins
Cook Time: 25 mins

Ingredients: 1 tsp olive oil, 4 chicken breast (sliced), 8 lettuce leaves (rinsed), 4 tbsp lemon juice (juice of 1 lemon), 4 tbsp cayenne pepper (try a drop of chili oil for extra heat), sea salt & fresh cracked pepper to taste.

Preparation:
-In a nonstick skillet over medium-high heat, add olive oil then sauté chicken for about 2 mins per side. Set aside.
-In the same skillet, add lemon juice and cayenne pepper (to taste) then bring to a boil. Add chicken back into the pan & turn down heat to 2 at a time (2 mins on each side). Serve immediately with lettuce leaf on top. Enjoy!

DINNER: **Beef Stew (low carb)**

Prep Time: 15 mins
Cook Time: 1 hr. 30 mins

Ingredients: 2 lbs. lean beef, 1 tbsp olive oil, 15oz can tomato sauce (undiluted), 2 tsp onion powder, 2 tsp garlic powder, 1/2 tsp oregano, 1/2 tsp dried basil, 3 tbsp Worcestershire sauce (low sodium), 1/4 cup red wine vinegar, 4 cups beef stock or water.

Preparation:

-In a large pot over medium heat, add oil then sauté beef for about 5 mins per side. Season with Worcestershire sauce and sea salt to taste. Set aside.
-In the same pot, add tomato sauce and season with onion powder, garlic powder, oregano and basil. Add in Worcestershire sauce and red wine vinegar then bring to a boil. Add in beef stock or water & bring to a simmer for about 30 mins until beef is tender (stir occasionally).
-Remove beef & set aside.
-In a blender, combine 1/2 of stew broth with Worcestershire sauce then blend (reserve the rest of broth). Heat up over medium heat then stir in the rest of stew broth (up to 8 cups). Season with sea salt & red pepper flakes to taste. Bring to a boil, then lower down heat to simmer for about 1 hr or until ready to serve.
-Divide stew evenly among large bowls then top with beef. Serve immediately.   Enjoy!

DAY 43

BREAKFAST: lasagna

Prep Time: 15 mins
Cook Time: 40 mins

Ingredients: 2 lasagna noodles (cooked), 1 onion (sliced), 1 capsicum (sliced), 3 tbsp olive oil, 4 eggs, 3 tomatoes (chopped), sea salt and fresh cracked pepper to taste.

Preparation:

-In a nonstick skillet over medium heat, add olive oil, sauté onions for about 5 mins, and capsicum and sauté for another 5 mins.   Set aside.
Preheat oven to 350 F. Lightly grease a medium-sized casserole dish with cooking spray or oil.   Add cooked lasagna noodles in the bottom of casserole dish then top with onion mixture. Layer with tomato and egg mixture then sprinkle with sea salt & fresh cracked pepper. Top with grated mozzarella cheese and bake for about 35 mins or until bubbly. Enjoy!

LUNCH: **Honey Mustard Salmon Wrap with Spinach, Carrots & Cucumber**

Prep Time: 15 mins
Cook Time: 20 mins

Ingredients: 1 salmon fillet (about 1lb), 1 tbsp olive oil, 8 lettuce leaves (rinsed), 3 tbsp honey mustard sauce, 4 carrots (shredded), 2 slices cucumber (diced), 2 cups spinach (chopped).

Preparation:
-In a medium pot, add water, then bring to a boil. Place salmon in the pot and cook for about 5 mins or until fish is cooked through. Remove from heat & set aside.   Let cool down (about 5 mins).
-In the same pot, add carrots, then cover with 2 cups of milk. Bring to a boil & cook for about 8 mins or until cooked through. Remove from heat & drain well (reserve milk).   Set aside
-Remove skin and bones from salmon & flake into small pieces.   In a large bowl, combine cooked salmon with cucumber & spinach then divide mixture evenly between lettuce leaves. Serve immediately.

DINNER: **Grilled Snapper with Sautéed Spinach & Garlic**

Prep Time: 15 mins
Cook Time: 25 mins

Ingredients: 1 snapper fillet (about 1lb), 1 tsp olive oil, 2 onions (sliced), sea salt and fresh cracked pepper to taste, 6 garlic cloves (minced). 1 bag of baby spinach leaves. 4 tbsp olive oil.

Preparation:
-In a large nonstick skillet over medium heat, add onions then sauté for about 5 mins then add snapper and season with sea salt & pepper to taste. Cook on each side for about 5 mins per side. Remove from heat & set aside.
-In the same skillet, add garlic then sauté for about 1 min or until fragrant. Add spinach and season with sea salt & pepper to taste. Sauté for another 3 mins or until wilted. Remove from heat & set aside.
-Preheat grill to medium-high heat (450 F). Preheat oil in a small bowl then drizzle over the chicken and spinach mixture.   Grill for approx. 3 mins & turn over to cook other side (be careful not to burn spinach). Serve immediately with cucumber slices on top if desired.
Enjoy!

DAY 44

BREAKFAST: Eggplant Parmesan

Prep Time: 15 mins
Cook Time: 45 mins

Ingredients: 1 eggplant (about 8), 1 cup mozzarella cheese (shredded), 4 tbsp butter, 1 cup parmesan cheese, sea salt & fresh cracked pepper to taste.

Preparation:
-Slice eggplant into ½-inch slices then put in a nonstick skillet over medium-high heat with sea salt & pepper and drizzle with olive oil. Sauté for about 10 mins or until eggplant starts to brown then turn off heat and let cool down.
Preheat oven to 350 F. Lightly grease a casserole dish with cooking spray or oil. Place eggplant slices on the bottom of the casserole dish then top with the shredded mozzarella & parmesan cheese. Bake for about 10 mins then remove from oven and let cool down for about 10 mins before serving (leave oven on). Enjoy!

LUNCH: Greek Omelet

Prep Time: 15 mins
Cook Time: 20 mins

Ingredients: 1 cup feta cheese (shredded), 1 can diced tomatoes & basil, 2 eggs (beaten), 1 tsp oregano, 3 tbsp olive oil, sea salt & pepper to taste.

Preparation:
-In a medium nonstick skillet over medium heat, add olive oil then sauté eggs for about 5 mins then remove from heat and set aside.
-In the same pan add feta cheese & season with sea salt & pepper to taste; then cook for about 5 mins or until browned then remove from heat and set aside. In a small bowl combine eggs with tomatoes & basil; add in oregano. Stir well before serving.

DINNER: Grilled Chicken with Cauliflower Salad

Prep Time: 15 mins
Cook Time: 15 mins

Ingredients: 1 whole chicken (about 2lb), 1 bag of baby spinach leaves, sea salt to taste, 1 cup olive oil. 2 tbsp dijon mustard, 3 tbsp honey mustard sauce.

Preparation:
-In a medium-sized nonstick skillet over medium-high heat, add olive oil, then sauté chicken for about 10 mins per side or until cooked through then remove from heat and let cool down.   Slice in half (breast half) and baste with honey mustard sauce then grill for about 4 mins on each side. Serve with cauliflower salad and dressing of your choice (Greek or honey mustard).

DAY 45

BREAKFAST: **Fettuccine Alfredo with chicken and broccoli**
Prep Time: 15 mins
Cook Time: 30 mins

Ingredients: 1 clove garlic (minced), 1 cup ricotta cheese, 2 cups spinach (chopped), 4 eggs, sea salt & pepper to taste, 2 chicken breasts (boneless and skinless), 1 cup fettuccine pasta, 3 cups broccoli florets.

Preparation:
-In a large nonstick skillet, combine 3 cups of water, sea salt & pepper and bring to a boil. Add pasta; cover and cook for about 8 mins or until cooked through. Cook chicken breast in the meantime (in a separate nonstick skillet over medium-high heat with some oil). Slice cooked chicken into thin strips and set aside (keep extra for another day).
Preheat oven to 350 F. Lightly grease a medium-sized casserole dish with cooking spray. Add broccoli to casserole dish, then layer with spinach & sauce mixture then top with pasta & chicken strips. Bake for about 10 mins or until heated through. Serve immediately with sour cream or plain yogurt on top if desired.

LUNCH: **Southwest Scrambled Eggs in a Tortilla with Salsa and Sour Cream**
Prep Time: 2 hours

Ingredients: 2 eggs (hard-boiled), 1 cup bell pepper (sliced), 1 onion (diced), 3 tbsp olive oil, 1 tsp cumin, sea salt & pepper to taste. 3 tbsp salsa, 1/2 cup sour cream.

Preparation:

-In a medium-sized nonstick skillet over medium-high heat, add oil, then sauté onion and bell pepper until onion is translucent (about 5 mins).   Add cumin then cook for another minute.

-In a medium-sized bowl, scramble eggs and season with sea salt & pepper to taste. Add in salsa then set aside.

Heat tortillas (I placed mine in the microwave for about 30 sec).   To assemble: add 2 tbsp of vegetable mixture to each tortilla, then top with 2 tbsp of the egg mixture and one slice of cheese (or more if desired).   Wrap and serve or eat open-faced like a wrap. Enjoy!

DINNER: **Roasted Asparagus and Chickpea Salad over Romaine Lettuce with a Creamy Lemon Dressing**

Prep Time: 20 mins
Cook Time: 15 mins

Ingredients: 1 cup canned chickpeas (drained & rinsed), 1 cup grape tomatoes, 2 cups asparagus (chopped), 1 cup spinach leaves (chopped), 3 tbsp olive oil, 2 tbsp lemon juice, sea salt & pepper to taste, 1/4 cup feta cheese (crumbled)

Preparation:

-In a small bowl whisk together olive oil, lemon juice and sea salt & pepper. Set aside.

-In a large nonstick skillet over medium-high heat, add olive oil, then sauté veggies until asparagus is tender (about 10 mins); set aside.

-Add cooked veggies to a large bowl then stir in feta cheese and lemon juice mixture. Serve over Romaine lettuce with some feta cheese crumbled on top if desired.
Enjoy!

DAY 46

BREAKFAST: **Pizza Margherita**

Prep Time: 20 mins
Cook Time: 15 mins

Ingredients: 1lb lean ground beef, sea salt & pepper to taste, 1/2 cup parmesan cheese (grated), 1 cup mozzarella cheese (grated), 1 tsp garlic powder, 6 sundried tomatoes (chopped), 1 large tomato (sliced), 3 eggs.

Preparation:
-In a large nonstick skillet over medium-high heat, add ground beef; season with salt & pepper to taste. Cook for about 10 mins or until cooked through, then remove from heat and set aside.   Heat oven to 425 F. -In a medium-sized bowl mix together all ingredients; set aside.
-In the same skillet over medium-high heat, add olive oil then saute eggs (in batches) until desired doneness. Serve with tomato slices on top if desired. Enjoy!

LUNCH: Spicy Turkey Sausage Patties with Eggs, Cheese and Tomato on an English Muffin

Prep Time: 10 mins
Cook Time: 15 mins
Ingredients: 1 package of ground turkey (9 oz), 2 eggs, 1/2 cup mozzarella cheese (shredded), 2 tbsp parsley (chopped), sea salt & pepper to taste, 1 clove garlic (minced)

Preparation:
-In a large nonstick skillet over medium-high heat, add some oil then sauté garlic for about 2 mins. Add turkey and season with salt & pepper to taste. Cook for about 5 mins or until cooked through, then remove from heat and set aside.
-In a small bowl mix together eggs, cheese & parsley then season with sea salt & pepper to taste. Set aside. -In the same skillet over medium-high heat, add olive oil then cook eggs quickly until desired doneness (sprinkle cheese on top after flipping each egg). Top each egg with turkey mixture and serve immediately.

DINNER: Bacon Wrapped Asparagus and Eggs

Prep Time: 10 mins
Cook Time: 30 mins

Ingredients: 12 slices (1 lb.) bacon, 1 lb. asparagus (chopped), sea salt, 4 eggs.

Preparation:
-In a large skillet over medium-high heat, add in chopped asparagus and sea salt to taste. Sauté for about 3 to 4 mins until asparagus is tender then set aside.
-In a large nonstick skillet over medium-high heat, add 1 tbsp olive oil then fry bacon (in batches) until crispy (about 5 mins).   Remove from heat and cut into large strips then set aside.
-In the same skillet over medium-high heat, add olive oil then cook scrambled eggs until desired doneness. Serve with bacon strips on top if desired.
Enjoy!

DAY 47

BREAKFAST: Quiche Lorraine

Prep Time: 15 mins
Cook Time: 40 mins

Ingredients: 16 slices bacon (cooked & crumbled), 2 cups mixed vegetables (chopped), 1 onion (diced), 1 clove garlic (minced), 4 eggs, 1 pie crust.

Preparation:

-In a large nonstick skillet over medium-high heat, add in onion & garlic then cook until translucent. Add mixed vegetables, stir for about 3 mins until cooked through, then set aside.
-In another large nonstick skillet over medium-high heat, add olive oil then sauté bacon until cooked through then remove from heat and set aside to cool slightly.
-In a large bowl, whisk together eggs, then add in vegetable mixture. Pour mixture into prepared crust then sprinkle with bacon.
Bake for about 40 mins at 350 F or until the center is set (you can also cook under the broiler for the last few minutes if desired).
-Serve warm with fruit and milk or yogurt.

LUNCH: Almond Breakfast Bars, Energy Bites or Baked Oatmeal Bar Cereal with Fruit & Milk or Yogurt

Prep Time: 10 mins
Cook Time: 15 mins

Ingredients: 2 squares (1/2 oz) almond butter (whipped), 1/3 cup honey (or other sweetener), 1/4 cup natural peanut butter, 3 tbsp coconut flour, 4 tbsp unsweetened shredded coconut, 1 tsp vanilla extract

Preparation:

-In a small bowl, whisk together honey & almond butter, then add peanut butter, coconut flour, and vanilla extract. Mix until incorporated then roll into 25 oz sized balls (or demitasse bars).
-In a large nonstick skillet, add some coconut oil over medium-high heat, then sauté demitasse bars until browned on all sides (about 5 mins). Place on a dish lined with parchment paper while you cook the rest.
-Serve with fruit and milk or yogurt.
Enjoy!

DINNER: **Green Bean & Tomato Salad with Toasted Almonds, Basil and Shallots on a Bed of Arugula**

Prep Time: 15 mins
Cook Time: 15 mins

Ingredients: 2 cups green beans (chopped), 1 cup tomato (sliced), 4 basil leaves (chopped), 1/2 cup almonds (slivered), 3 tbsp olive oil, 2 tsp balsamic vinegar, sea salt & pepper to taste.

Preparation:

-In a large nonstick skillet over medium-high heat, add olive oil then sauté green beans for about 1 min. Season with salt & pepper to taste then set aside.
-In the same skillet over medium-high heat, add sliced tomatoes, then cook for about 5 mins or until cooked through. Set aside. -In the same skillet over medium-high heat, add olive oil then sauté basil, almonds and sea salt to taste just until cooked through (about 3 mins).   Set aside.
-In a large mixing bowl, toss together beans and tomato then serve immediately with slivered almonds on top.   Top with balsamic vinegar if desired.
Enjoy!

DAY 48

BREAKFAST: **Salmon with asparagus and brown rice**

Prep Time: 15 mins
Cook Time: 25 mins

Ingredients: 2 cups brown rice (cooked), 1/2 tsp ground ginger, 1/4 tsp garlic powder, 1/4 cup fresh chopped asparagus (1 stalk), sea salt & pepper to taste, 1 small salmon fillet (about 4 oz).

Preparation:

-In a nonstick skillet over medium-high heat, add olive oil then add in asparagus and cook until just tender. Season with sea salt & pepper to taste then set aside.
-In the same skillet over medium-high heat, add in salmon fillets and season with sea salt & pepper to taste. Cook for about 6 to 8 mins depending on thickness of fillet or until cooked through, then set aside.
-In a small bowl, season rice with ground ginger, garlic powder & sea salt to taste then place in a serving dish along with asparagus.   Spoon salmon and cooking juices on top and serve.
Enjoy!

LUNCH: **Strawberry Pancakes with the Taste of Summer**

Prep Time: 10 mins
Cook Time: 15 mins

Ingredients 4 slices bacon (cooked & crumbled), 4 tbsp coconut flour, 4 tbsp butter (melted), 1/4 cup + 1 tbsp honey, 2 eggs, 1/2 tsp baking soda, 1 cup strawberries (sliced).

Preparation:

-In a large nonstick skillet over medium-high heat, add bacon, then cook for about 3 mins or until cooked through. Remove from heat and set aside.

-In the same skillet over medium-high heat, add butter, then whisk in honey & coconut flour until incorporated. Whisk in eggs then pour mixture into pancake batter maker (or food processor). Follow directions on machine or mix by hand until well combined. Place into a heated pan and spread-out pancake batter evenly in the pan (about 2 inches).

-Top with sliced strawberries and serve warm sprinkled with crumbled bacon.
Enjoy!

DINNER: **Grilled Chicken with Spinach and Bell Pepper Couscous**

Prep Time: 10 mins
Cook Time: 30 min

Ingredients: 1 cup couscous (cooked), 1 tbsp olive oil, 2 tomatoes, 1 cucumber (chopped), 1/2 bell pepper, 2 chicken breasts (boneless & skinless), 3 cups baby spinach leaves.

Preparation:

-Season chicken breasts with sea salt & pepper to taste, then grill on each side for about 6 to 8 minutes or until cooked through.

-In a small bowl, whisk together olive oil and lemon juice then pour over couscous to easily rinse off excess oil. Place couscous into a serving dish covered with foil and set aside.

-In the same skillet over medium-high heat, add tomatoes, then season with sea salt & pepper to taste just until heated through (about 1 min). Add in cucumber & bell pepper & cook until tender (about 3 mins). Season chicken breast with sea salt & black pepper to taste then place on top of vegetables and serve warm.

DAY 49

BREAKFAST: **Classic Meatloaf**

Prep Time: 15 mins
Cook Time: 45 mins

Ingredients: 2 lbs. ground beef (ground pork, turkey or chicken), 1 egg (lightly beaten), salt & pepper to taste.

Preparation:
-In a large mixing bowl, combine beef and egg, then season with salt & pepper to taste. Mix well then form into a loaf shape and place on a baking dish that's lined with foil. Bake at 375 degrees F for about 45 mins or until cooked through. Serve warm topped with some Cheetos if desired.

LUNCH: **Egg & Cheddar Quiche with Mixed Vegetables**

Prep Time: 10 mins
Cook Time: 30 mins

Ingredients: 1 large egg (lightly beaten), 1/4 cup shredded cheddar cheese (divided), salt & pepper to taste, 2 tbsp olive oil, 1 small onion (chopped).

Preparation:
-In a small bowl, combine egg and cheese then season with sea salt & pepper to taste. Set aside.
-Whisk together egg and cheese mixture until well combined then in a nonstick skillet over medium-high heat, add olive oil, add onion, and cook for about 5 minutes or until tender. Set aside.
-In an ungreased baking dish, spread egg mixture then spread onion mixture on top. Bake at 375 degrees F for about 20 mins or until cooked through. Enjoy!

DINNER: **Roasted Cauliflower and Pear Salad**

Prep Time: 10 mins
Cook Time: 40 mins

Ingredients: 2 cups cauliflower (chopped), 3 tsp olive oil, salt & pepper to taste, 1 pear (sliced), 1 cup spinach.

Preparation:
-Place cauliflower in a small mixing bowl, then drizzle with olive oil and season with sea salt & pepper to taste. Toss & toss to evenly coat, then spread onto a large baking sheet that's lined with

foil. Place into oven on a rack position about 6 to 8 inches away from the heat source. Roast for about 30 mins or until tender and slightly browned on top.

-In a large mixing bowl, combine cauliflower, spinach and pear then season with sea salt & pepper to taste. Top with additional cheddar cheese if desired & serve warm drizzled with olive oil.

Enjoy!

DAY 50

BREAKFAST: Spaghetti Carbonara with Chicken and Mushrooms

Prep Time: 5 mins
Cook Time: 10 mins

Ingredients: 1 tsp olive oil, 3 slices of bacon (cooked), 4 oz shiitake mushrooms, 1 small chicken breast (about 4 oz).

Preparation:

-In a nonstick skillet over medium-high heat, add in oil, add in bacon, then cook for about 3 mins or until cooked through. Remove from heat & set aside. -In the same skillet over medium-high heat, add in mushrooms & chicken breast then season with sea salt & pepper to taste. Cook for about 6 to 8 mins or until cooked through, then set aside. -In a small bowl, whisk together half & half & 1 egg, pour into the same skillet, and then add in cooked noodles. Cook for about 5 mins or until sauce thickens and noodles are tender, then sprinkle with crumbled bacon and serve warm. Enjoy!

LUNCH: Southwest Wraps

Prep Time: 10 mins
Cook Time: 15 mins

Ingredients: 2 large lettuce leaves, 1 small tomato (sliced), 3 slices cheese (any kind), 3 oz cooked ground beef, 3 tbsp guacamole (homemade or store-bought), 2 tbsp sour cream, 1/4 cup onion (chopped).

Preparation:

-In a small bowl, mash guacamole with a fork then stir in sour cream until combined. Set aside.
-In a large tortilla, add lettuce and then a layer of tomato slices (do not stack). Top with cheese then ground beef (if desired) then add more lettuce and tomatoes if needed. Top with onion and guacamole & serve warm.

DINNER: Grilled Pork Loin with Sweet Potatoes and Pear Salsa over Quinoa

Prep Time: 15 mins
Cook Time: 25 mins

Ingredients: 1/2 cup quinoa (cooked & cooled), 2 cups sweet potatoes (cooked, peeled & diced), 3 large pears (diced), 1 tsp cinnamon, salt & pepper to taste, 2 tbsp olive oil.

Preparation:
-In a medium mixing bowl, season pork with sea salt & pepper to taste, then place in a large skillet over medium heat. Cook on all sides for about 7 to 9 mins or until cooked through.
-In the same skillet over medium-high heat, add in oil, then add in pears and cook for about 4 to 5 mins or until tender. Add in quinoa and cinnamon then stir until combined and warm. Season with sea salt & pepper to taste then serve warm as it is or top with chopped pecans if desired. Enjoy!

DAY 51

BREAKFAST: Chicken Noodle Soup

Prep Time: 10 mins
Cook Time: 30-45 mins

Ingredients: 1 small onion (chopped), 2 cloves garlic (minced), 2 celery stalks (chopped), 1/2 tsp paprika, salt & pepper to taste.

Preparation:
-In a large pot over medium heat, add in onion then sauté for about 7 to 8 mins or until tender. Add in garlic and cook for about 1 min or until lightly browned. Stir in celery & paprika, then season with sea salt & pepper to taste.
-Stir well, add in chicken stock/broth and boil. Reduce heat so that it's simmering, then cover with lid & simmer for about 30 mins or until cooked through. Add more of the chicken broth if needed before serving.
-In a medium mixing bowl, whisk together eggs, then season with sea salt & pepper to taste. Pour into the same skillet, then add in cooked noodles and cheese (if desired) and stir until well combined. Top with scallions (optional) and serve warm.

LUNCH: **Veggie Frittata with Melted Feta and Spinach**

Prep Time: 10 mins
Cook Time: 30 mins

Ingredients: 1 large egg (lightly beaten), 2 tbsp olive oil, 1 small onion (chopped), 2 cloves garlic (minced), 1 cup spinach, salt & pepper to taste, 2 tbsp feta cheese (crumbled).

Preparation:
-In a large nonstick skillet over medium-high heat, add in oil, then add in onion and sauté for about 5 to 6 mins or until tender. Add in garlic and spinach, stir until wilted then reduce heat to low.
-In a small bowl, whisk together eggs and season with sea salt & pepper to taste. Pour eggs into the same skillet, then top with crumbled feta cheese (if desired) & serve warm.

DINNER: **Salmon Burgers with Avocado, Tomato & Cucumber on a Bed of Spinach with Low Carb Tortilla Chips**

Prep Time: 15 mins
Cook Time: 20 mins

Ingredients: 1 cup salmon (cooked & flaked), 3 tbsp onions (minced), salt & pepper to taste, 1 tbsp parsley (chopped), 2 tbsp olive oil, 2 slices cheese (any kind).

Preparation:
-In a medium mixing bowl, combine salmon with onions, salt & pepper to taste then add in parsley.   Form into 4 patties then place on a plate then set aside.
-In a large nonstick skillet over medium-high heat, add in oil and then add in patties then cook for about 5 to 6 mins per side or until cooked through. Serve on a bed of spinach (cooked & cooled) with garnished with sliced tomato and low-carb tortilla chips. Enjoy!

DAY 53

BREAKFAST: **Vegetarian Lentil Stew with Sweet Potatoes, Carrots, and Parsley**

Prep Time: 5 mins
Cook Time: 60 mins

Ingredients: 3 medium sweet potatoes (cooked & peeled), 2 cups baby carrots (cooked & sliced), 1 lb ground beef or turkey (cooked & crumbled), 1/4 cup onion (minced), 1/4 cup celery (minced), salt & pepper to taste.

Preparation:

-In a blender, combine all ingredients and blend until smooth, then spread evenly in a large skillet over medium heat. Cook for about 15 to 20 mins or until sauce is thickened. Serve warm over top of cooked quinoa.

LUNCH: **Cauliflower Pizza Bagels**

Prep Time: 10 mins
Cook Time: 15-20 mins

Ingredients: 2 large head cauliflower (cut into florets), 2 cups pine nuts (lightly toasted), 1 medium head garlic (or 6 cloves, minced or pressed), salt & pepper to taste, 1 small zucchini (diced), 1 small yellow squash (diced).

Preparation:

-In a food processor, pulse together cauliflower florets & pine nuts for about 3 minutes or until well chopped. Add in garlic & pulse for a few seconds more. Season with salt & pepper to taste.
Preheat oven to 425 degrees F. Line a baking sheet with parchment paper, spread cauliflower mixture onto the lined baking sheet, forming into 4 large circular patties. Bake for about 15 mins or until crisped around the edges. Meanwhile, in a large skillet over medium-high heat, add in zucchini and yellow squash, then cook until tender but still firm, stirring frequently (about 10 mins). Remove from heat and set aside. Remove patties from oven then top each with zucchini & squash mixture and serve.

DINNER: **Smoky Balsamic Steak with Eggplant & Zucchini over Quinoa**

Prep Time: 30 mins
Cook Time: 30-40 mins

Ingredients: 1 lb. flank steak (cooked), 1 tbsp olive oil, 1 medium zucchini (cut in half and sliced), 2 large eggplants (sliced into thick rounds), salt & pepper to taste.

Preparation:

-In a large skillet over medium heat, add in steak and then cook for about 7 mins per side or until desired doneness. Set aside.

-Add the same skillet over medium heat, then add in oil and cook eggplant rounds, turning once (about 10 to 15 mins). Season with salt & pepper to taste.

Preheat oven to 350 degrees F. In a large baking dish, arrange vegetables as shown in the picture, then top with steak. Roast for about 20 mins or until vegetables are tender. Remove from oven and serve hot over top of quinoa. Enjoy!

DAY 53

BREAKFAST: Autumn Squash Risotto

Prep Time: 5 mins
Cook Time: 30 mins

Ingredients: 1 cup butternut squash (cubed), 2 cups arborio rice (cooked), 4 cups chicken broth, 1/4 cup onion (chopped), salt & pepper to taste.

Preparation:

-In a large saucepan over medium-high heat, add in cubed squash, then cook for about 5 mins or until softened. -Reduce heat to medium, add rice, stir well to combine.
-Pour in chicken broth and cook for about 20 mins or until liquid has been absorbed.
-Stir occasionally and season with salt & pepper to taste.
-Serve & enjoy!

LUNCH: Pennsylvania Dutch Hot Dish with Turkey, Peppers & Onions

Prep Time: 10 mins
Cook Time: 20-30 mins

Ingredients: 2 lbs. ground turkey, 1 large onion (chopped), 1 large green bell pepper (diced), 1/2 cup celery (diced), 1 cup cooked long grain brown rice, salt & pepper to taste.

Preparation:

-In a large skillet, brown turkey over medium-high heat, then remove and set aside.
-Dice onion, pepper and celery then return same skillet to medium-high heat and sauté for about 5 mins until onions are translucent and celery is tender. Add back in turkey along with cooked rice & salt & pepper to taste. Stir while frying until well combined, then cook for about 20 mins or until warmed through. Serve & enjoy!

DINNER: Sausage, Mushroom and Leek Manicotti

Prep Time: 15 mins
Cook Time: 25 mins

Ingredients: 1 lb. ground pork sausage, 4-5 whole eggs (beaten), 4 ounces cream cheese, 1/2 cup mozzarella cheese (shredded), 1 bunch (about 10) whole leeks (sliced in half & washed thoroughly), 1 tsp parsley (chopped), salt & pepper to taste.

Preparation:

-In a large mixing bowl, combine all ingredients then form into 12 large ovals. Set aside.
-In a large saucepan over medium-high heat, add in olive oil then add in leeks & season with salt & pepper to taste. Cook for about 10 mins, then remove and set aside.
-Pour off any excess oil left in the pan, then add in ovals and cook for about 10 mins per side or until golden brown and cooked through. Serve with roasted asparagus (lightly seasoned with salt).

DAY 54

BREAKFAST: Apple Crisp

Prep Time: 10 mins
Cook Time: 35 mins

Ingredients: 4 medium apples (peeled & sliced), 1 cup oats (quick cooking), 1/4 cup whole wheat pastry flour, 3 tbsp cold butter, 2 tbsp white sugar (divided), 1.5 tsp cinnamon, 3 tbsp brown sugar, salt & pepper to taste.

Preparation:

-Set aside butter for later then in a large saucepan over medium heat, add remaining ingredients and stir well. Cook for about 8 mins or until apples are soft but still hold their shape. Remove from heat, spread evenly into a large baking dish, and set aside.
Preheat oven to 350 degrees F, then put butter back in the pan over medium-high heat with 1 tbsp of brown sugar and mix well till melted. Pour over top of apples & bake for about 15 mins or until bubbly around the edges (oven temps vary so watch closely). Remove from oven & serve warm with whipped cream.

LUNCH: **Veggie Scrambled Egg Burrito**

Prep Time: 5 mins

Ingredients: 1 large egg (beaten), 1/4 cup cheddar cheese (shredded), 1/4 cup avocado (pureed), pinch salt, pinch pepper.

Preparation:

-In a small bowl, combine all ingredients then set aside.

-Heat a large skillet over medium-high heat, crack in egg, and cook for about 2 mins or until scrambled. Keep scrambled egg in the same skillet.

-Unwrap burrito sized tortilla and place on the counter then spoon on half of the scrambled egg mix and roll into burrito form. Secure with toothpick if needed. Place on a plate and repeat with remaining ingredients. Serve with salsa and sliced avocados.

DINNER: **Grilled Pork Chops with Cauliflower Mash**

Prep Time: 5 mins

Ingredients: 16 oz pork chops (sliced in half), 1/2 cup cheddar cheese (shredded), 1 cup spinach, 1/4 cup scallions (chopped), salt & pepper to taste.

Preparation:

Preheat grill pan over medium-high heat, add pork chops to grill pan, and cook for about 5 mins per side or until desired doneness. (The thinner the better, so be sure to slice pork chops in half horizontally).

-While pork chops are cooking, place all other ingredients in a food processor and mix till it's texture of mashed potatoes. Season with salt & pepper to taste.

Preheat oven to 350 degrees F then spread over cauliflower mix on top of sliced cheddar cheese then place in oven and bake for about 10 mins or until cheese has melted on top and cauliflower is cooked through.

Serve & enjoy!

DAY 55

BREAKFAST: **Pumpkin Spice Pancakes with Maple Syrup**

Prep Time: 10 mins

Cook Time: 15 mins

Ingredients: 3/4 cup whole wheat pastry flour, 1/2 tsp baking powder, 1 tbsp brown sugar, 1/2 tsp cinnamon, pinch salt, 2 large eggs (separated), 1 cup butternut squash (cubed and cooked), 2 tbsp coconut oil or olive oil.

Preparation:

-In a medium mixing bowl, combine whole wheat flour and baking powder, then mix in brown sugar and cinnamon. Set aside.

Preheat a large skillet over medium-high heat, then add coconut oil and cubed butternut squash. Cook for about 5 mins or until squash is tender, then remove from pan and set aside.

-In the same pan, add in olive oil then stir in egg yolks then cook for about 1 min or until bubbly on top. -Add flour mixture and stir well to coat along with squash, then cook for about 1 min more. Remove from heat and let cool slightly. -In a large mixing bowl, combine egg whites, vanilla extract and maple syrup then whisk till foamy. Fold into whole mix and cook on the skillet over medium-high heat for 3 mins per side or until golden brown & cooked through (the thinner the better so watch closely). -Serve warm with maple syrup.

LUNCH: **Southwest Chicken Wrap with Salsa & Sour Cream on a Whole Wheat Tortilla**

Prep Time: 5 mins

Ingredients: 1/4 cup salsa (homemade or store-bought), 1/4 cup sour cream, 1 large whole wheat tortilla, 3 oz grilled chicken breast (thin sliced), salt & pepper to taste.

Preparation:

-Spread the sour cream evenly over one-half the tortilla, then top with salsa and chicken slices. Fold over then secure with toothpick if needed. Place on plate and repeat with the other half of the tortilla and desired ingredients. -Heat a large skillet over medium heat, then pour in coconut oil and add in chicken to pan. Cook for about 3 mins or until desired doneness (thinner not cooked through, so watch closely). Remove from pan and set aside.

-Pour off all oil left in pan, add unwrapped tortillas, and fill with chicken, spinach leaves, etc. Place pan back on heat, then pour 1 tbsp of salsa and stir well to coat. Remove from heat and serve.

DINNER: **Cauliflower Fried Rice**

Prep Time: 5 mins

Ingredients: 1 head cauliflower (cut into small florets), 3 eggs (beaten), 2 tbsp soy sauce, 1/4 cup green onions (chopped), salt & pepper to taste.

Preparation:

-Steam cauliflower over medium-high heat for about 15 mins, then set aside. -In the meantime, heat a large skillet over medium-high heat then add in olive oil, bacon and stir for about 4 mins or until bacon is cooked. Remove from pan and set aside. -In the same pan, pour in soy sauce and stir well to coat along with eggs, then add green onions. Cook for about 1 min or until egg is cooked through on bottom (the thinner the better so watch closely). Set aside while cooking cauliflower rice. -Add in cauliflower rice and sautéed bacon and mix well to coat along with salt & pepper to taste. -Serve.

DAY 56

BREAKFAST: **Rosemary Roasted Potatoes and Brussels Sprouts with Shallots**

Prep Time: 10 mins
Cook Time: 35 mins

Ingredients: 1/4 cup olive oil, 4 cloves garlic (minced), 2 lb. fingerling baby potatoes (halved), 1 lb. brussels sprouts (halved), 1/4 cup rosemary leaves, salt & pepper to taste.

Preparation:

-Preheat oven to 425 degrees F, then line a baking sheet with parchment paper and drizzle over olive oil then place shallots and garlic on top. Season with salt & pepper to taste, then mix well.
-Roast for 10 mins then add in Brussels sprouts and potatoes and mix again. Roast for about 35 mins more or until potatoes are tender and golden brown. -Serve warm.

LUNCH: **Tuna Salad, Chicken Salad or Ham & Cheese (with lettuce) in Pita Bread**

Prep Time: 10 mins
Cook Time: 25 mins

Ingredients: 1/2 cup tuna (canned), 1/2 cup cooked chicken breast, 1/2 cup ham (diced), 1/2 cup bacon (diced), 2 tbsp crumbled feta cheese, 1 tsp olive oil, 2 tbsp mayonnaise, salt & pepper to taste.

Preparation:

-In a bowl, combine all ingredients, then season to taste. Keeps in fridge for 3 days or freeze. -Place pitas flat on a baking sheet and place in oven for about 2 mins each side or until warm. -Remove from oven then top with lettuce & desired toppings then serve.

DINNER: **Grilled Chicken Caesar Salad over Creamy Lemon Chicken Wrap with Romaine Lettuce & Bacon**

Prep Time: 10 mins

Ingredients: 1/2 cup lemon juice, 2 cloves garlic (minced), 2 tbsp olive oil, 2 tbsp capers, 4 cans chicken breast (cut in small strips), 4 romaine and spinach leaves (sliced thin), salt & pepper to taste.

Preparation:

-In a bowl, stir together lemon juice and garlic then set aside. -Heat a large skillet over medium-high heat, add olive oil and sauté chicken breast, then season with salt & pepper to taste. Remove from pan and set aside. -In the same pan, pour in lemon juice mixture and capers then cook for about 2 mins more or until sauce thickens. -Place chicken back in pan once again along with spinach, romaine lettuce and mix well till coated along with salt & pepper to taste. -Serve warm.

DAY 57

BREAKFAST: **Italian Bruschetta Salad**

Prep Time: 10 mins
Cook Time: 10 mins

Ingredients: 1/2 cup fresh basil leaves (chopped), 1/2 cup roasted red peppers (halved, seeded and chopped), 1/2 cup sliced onion (chopped) 2 tbsp olive oil, 1 tsp each salt & pepper, 1 garlic clove (crushed).

Preparation:

-In a bowl, combine all ingredients, then season to taste. Keeps in fridge for up to three days or freeze. -Serve with desired toppings (avocado is great too!).

LUNCH: **Egg, Mushroom and Cheese in a Pita Pocket or Wraps**

Prep Time: 5 mins

Ingredients: 1 large eggplant (cut into small rounds), 1/4 cup olive oil, 2 oz mushrooms (sliced), 1/4 cup green onions (chopped), mayonnaise, salt & pepper to taste, 2 pita pockets.

Preparation:
-Place eggplant slices on a baking sheet and drizzle over olive oil then season with salt & pepper to taste then roast in the oven at 400 degrees F for about 10 mins or until soft.
-In the meantime, heat a large skillet over medium-high heat, then add in olive oil and sauté mushrooms until they soften. Season with salt & pepper to taste then set aside.
-Spread 1 tbsp of mayonnaise inside each pita pocket along with some roasted eggplant rounds, mushrooms and chopped green onions.
-Serve warm or cold.

DINNER: Paleo Meatballs (vegan, low carb)
Prep Time: 5 mins

Ingredients: 2 eggs (beaten), 1/4 cup parsley (chopped), 1 garlic clove (minced), 1.5 tbsp each oregano, basil and marjoram in a bowl then season with salt & pepper to taste.

Preparation:
-In a bowl, mix all ingredients well, then form into balls, place on a sprayed baking dish or perforated pan, and place in oven at 350 degrees F for 30 mins or until cooked through.
-Sprinkle with desired toppings of choice(s). Serve warm.

DAY 58

BREAKFAST: Southwest Steak Salad
Prep Time: 5 mins
Cook Time: 10 mins

Ingredients: 1 cup baby spinach leaves, 1/2 cup black beans (drained and rinsed), 1/4 cup avocado cubes, 2 oz cooked steak (cut into chunks), salt & pepper to taste.

Preparation:
-In a bowl, place spinach and beans, then season with salt & pepper to taste, then mix well.
-In a large skillet over medium heat, add avocado cubes, steak, and salt & pepper to taste.
-Let mixture cook for about 2 mins until heated through. Stir well then serve warm.

LUNCH: **Ham & Cheese Sloppy Joes**

Prep Time: 5 mins
Cook Time: 10 mins

Ingredients: 1/2 cup diced ham (shredded), 2 tbsp white onion (minced), 2 slices of cheese (shredded).

Preparation:

-In a bowl, combine all ingredients, then season with salt & pepper to taste.
-Place in a skillet over medium heat and cook for about 3-5 mins or until cheese melts.
-Serve warm.

DINNER: **Paleo Beef Stew (vegan, low carb)**

Prep Time: 5 mins
Cook Time: 40 mins

Ingredients: 1 1/2 lb. beef stew meat (sliced into 1/4-inch strips), 3 carrots (cut into large chunks), 2 celery stalks (cut into pieces), 1 onion (chopped), 2 tbsp olive oil, 2 bay leaves, 1 tsp each oregano and rosemary in a bowl then season with salt & pepper to taste.

Preparation:

-In a bowl, stir together olive oil and seasonings then coat beef slices with mixture.
-Place a large pot over medium heat then add in beef, onions, carrots, and salt & pepper to taste. Sauté for about 4 mins. -Pour in enough water to cover, then bring to a boil until veggies are tender & meat is cooked through. Remove from heat once done then add in celery and bay leaves. Let cool then skim off excess fat before serving warm.
-Serve with desired toppings of choice.

DAY 59

BREAKFAST: **Chicken Quesadilla**

Prep Time: 10 mins
Cook Time: 10 mins

Ingredients: 1/2 cup chopped onion (diced), 1 tbsp olive oil, 1 clove garlic (minced), 3oz chicken breast (cooked & diced), 2 tbsp salsa, tortilla, salt & pepper to taste.

Preparation:

-In a pan over medium heat, add in olive oil and sauté chicken breast, then season with salt & pepper to taste. -In a small bowl, mix salsa with onion and garlic then set aside. -On a large tortilla, layer chicken, salsa and onions, then season with salt & pepper to taste. Roll tortilla up and place on a sprayed baking dish or perforated pan along with sprayed top down. -Bake at 400 degrees F for about 10 mins or until tortilla gets nice golden-brown crispiness on top. -Serve warm.

LUNCH: Grilled Chicken & Veggies, with Avocado Salsa & Medium Buns

Prep Time: 5 mins
Cook Time: 15 mins

Ingredients: 2 boneless skinless chicken breasts (sliced into thin strips), 1/4 cup olive oil, 3 green onions (sliced), 4 medium scallions (sliced), 2 tsp each oregano, salt & pepper to taste.

Preparation:

-In a bowl, combine olive oil and seasonings, then coat chicken until well coated.
-Heat a large skillet over medium-high heat then add in chicken along with seasonings. Cook for about 8 mins or until cooked through, then set aside to rest. Once cool, slice into strips.
-Add veggies to the same pan (without cleaning) over medium heat and sauté for about 4 mins or until tender-crisp, then set aside to rest.
-To assemble, place 3 slices of bread on a cutting board along with 2 avocado halves and scoop of beef stew if desired.
-Place grilled chicken and veggies in between which will act as your buns then enjoy.

DINNER: Basmati Rice & Lentils with Spinach (low carb)

Prep Time: 5 mins
Cook Time: 15 mins

Ingredients: 1/2 cup lentils (rinsed & drained), 2 cups water, 1.5 tbsp olive oil, kosher salt & pepper to taste, 1.5 cups basmati rice (cooked), 1 cup spinach (chopped).

Preparation:

-In a pan over medium heat, combine lentils and water then season with salt & pepper to taste. Let cook for about 10 mins or until tender.
-While the lentil mixture cooks, place rice in a bowl and drizzle over olive oil, then season with salt & pepper to taste, then toss well to coat evenly.
-Plate rice then top with lentils and spinach. Enjoy.

DAY 60

BREAKFAST: Grilled Chicken with Couscous and Feta

Prep Time: 5 mins
Cook Time: 10 mins

Ingredients: 1/4 cup olive oil, 8 oz cooked chicken breast (shredded), 1/4 cup feta cheese (crumbled), 2 tbsp olive oil, 2 cups cooked couscous, salt & pepper to taste.

Preparation:

-In a bowl, combine olive oil and seasonings then toss with chicken until well coated.
Preheat a grill over medium-high heat then place chicken on grill to cook for about 3-4 mins per side or until cooked through. Set aside to rest for a few minutes before slicing into strips then set aside.
-In a small bowl, drizzle over 2 tablespoons of olive oil to coat, then stir in feta cheese and mix well. Set aside for later use along with 1/2 cup couscous that has been separated from the other 1/2 cup (packaged together). -Plate 1/2 cup of remaining seasoned couscous, spoon over chicken strips, and drizzle feta cheese mixture evenly over top.
-Serve warm with desired toppings of choice.

LUNCH: Buffalo Chicken Salad

Prep Time: 10 mins
Cook Time: 10 mins

Ingredients: 3/4 cup Romaine lettuce (chopped), 2 oz cooked chicken breast (shredded), 1 celery stalk (sliced), 1 medium carrot (diced), 3 green onions (sliced), 2 tbsp light ranch dressing, 2 cups baby spinach leaves, salt & pepper to taste, 2 tbsp sliced almonds.

Preparation:

-In a large bowl, combine lettuce along with seasonings and toss until well coated.
Set aside. -In a separate bowl, combine chicken with celery and carrots, then season with salt & pepper to taste, then toss well to coat evenly. Set aside.
-In a small bowl, mix ranch dressing then toss with spinach leaves until well coated.
-Place spinach in the middle of the lettuce mix then top with chicken strips and celery/carrot mixture along with sliced almonds on top. Drizzle with 2 tablespoons of ranch dressing to finish.
-Serve chilled

DINNER: Cheddar Popper Burgers with Bacon Ketchup over Romaine Lettuce with a Side Salad & Zucchini Fries

Prep Time: 15 mins
Cook Time: 15 mins

Ingredients: 18 burger patties (1/4 inch thick), 1 cup shredded cheddar cheese, 2 tbsp bacon ketchup, 1/4 cup chopped basil, 4 cups baby spinach leaves, oil for frying.

Preparation:
-Heat oil in deep fryer over medium-high heat then add in patties and cook for about 4 mins on each side or until cooked through. Set aside to rest, then slice into strips.
-In a small bowl, mix bacon ketchup with basil then season with salt & pepper to taste.
-To assemble, place 2 slices of romaine lettuce on a plate, then top with 2 patties, about 1/4 cup of cheese and cut into 4 wedges.
-Serve with desired toppings of choice for sides.

DAY 61

BREAKFAST: Greek Salad

Prep Time: 5 mins
Cook Time: 15 mins

Ingredients: 1/4 cup olive oil, 2 pints grape tomatoes (halved), 2 cups arugula (packed), 1/2 cup feta cheese (crumbled), 2 tbsp Kalamata olives with pits, 1/4 cup Kalamata olives with pits & stems, salt & pepper to taste.

Preparation:
-In a bowl, combine olive oil with seasonings, toss with grape tomatoes, and set aside.
-In another bowl, combine arugula with seasonings and toss until well coated.
-To assemble, place a salad of your choice in the middle of 2 plates then top each plate with 1/2 cup of salad and 1 tbsp feta cheese. Drizzle over 2 tbsp of olive oil, then top each plate with remaining arugula and olives by alternating on both plates so that the olives are layered across each plate evenly. Enjoy!

LUNCH: **Chicken Caesar Salad**

Prep Time: 5 mins
Cook Time: 5 mins

Ingredients: 2 cups cooked chicken breast (shredded), 1 cup romaine lettuce (chopped), 1/2 cup Parmesan cheese (grated), 4 tbsp chopped basil, 2 tbsp olive oil from the salad dressing, 1/3 cup bottled Caesar dressing.

Preparation:
-In a small bowl, mix Caesar dressing with 2 tablespoons of olive oil then set aside for later use.
-In a large bowl, combine your lettuce with the remaining 3 tablespoons of oil then toss until well coated. -To assemble, place in the middle of 2 plates then top with chicken and sprinkle with Parmesan cheese. Drizzle over dressing and garnish with basil. Enjoy!

DINNER: **Spaghetti Squash Almondine (vegan, low carb)**

Prep Time: 10 mins
Cook Time: 15 mins

Ingredients: 2/3 cup flour, 1/2 cup almond meal, 1/4 tsp garlic powder, 1/4 tsp onion powder, 1 tsp paprika, salt & pepper to taste, olive oil for frying.

Preparation:
-In a bowl, combine flour, almond meal, and seasonings then season well.
-Add in paprika, salt and pepper to taste. -Heat oil in a pot over medium-high heat, then toss in your mixture until well coated. Reduce heat to medium, then cover and cook for about 4 mins or until almondine has browned slightly.
-Remove from heat, let cool then slice into almondine sticks.   Enjoy!

DAY 62

BREAKFAST: **Grilled Shrimp & Lemon Rice**

Prep Time: 10 mins
Cook Time: 15 mins

Ingredients: 6 medium shrimp (peeled & deveined), 1/2 cup uncooked white rice, 1 tsp olive oil, 2 tbsp chopped parsley, salt & pepper to taste.

Preparation:

-Stick a grill pan over medium high heat, then drizzle with olive oil and sauté shrimp for 2-3 mins each side or until cooked through.   Set aside to rest for a few minutes before slicing into strips then set aside.

-In a small bowl, combine seasonings to rice, then toss until well coated.

-Meanwhile, heat oil in a skillet over medium-high heat, add rice mixture, and cook for about 7 mins or until rice has browned slightly.

-Remove from heat, let cool then top with shrimp when ready to serve.

Enjoy!

LUNCH: **Southwest Egg Salad**

Prep Time: 5 mins
Cook Time: 5 mins

Ingredients: 1 hardboiled egg (chopped), 2 tbsp frozen corn, 1/2 cup canned black beans (rinsed & drained), 2 tbsp salsa, salt & pepper to taste, 1/2 cup spinach leaves.

Preparation:

-In a bowl, combine all ingredients except spinach leaves, then season with salt and pepper to taste.

-Serve over fresh spinach leaves as desired.

Enjoy!

DINNER: **Sweet Potato Fries & Avocado Dip or Guacamole (vegan, low carb)**

Prep Time: 5 mins
Cook Time: 10 mins

Ingredients: 4 medium sweet potatoes (peeled & chopped into strips), 1/4 cup avocado (mashed), salt & pepper to taste, 1 tsp olive oil, 3 tbsp cilantro.

Preparation:

-Combine avocado, yogurt, cilantro, garlic and lime juice in a blender then blend until well combined.

-In a skillet over medium heat, sauté sweet potato with olive oil and seasonings for about 10 mins or until fries are cooked through and well coated with spices. Remove from heat then set aside to cool.

-To assemble, place in the center of a plate and top with avocado dip. Enjoy!

DAY 63

BREAKFAST: Italian Sausage Cabbage Roll Soup

Prep Time: 10 mins
Cook Time: 15 mins

Ingredients: 1/4 lb. Italian Sausage (cut into rings), 2 -6 cups cabbage (shredded then cooked), 1 tbsp olive oil, 3 cloves garlic, 1 cup green onions (chopped), 4 cups tomato sauce, salt & pepper to taste.

Preparation:
-In a large pot, brown sausage in oil over medium-high heat, then remove from heat and set aside.
-In the same pot, add garlic, onions, and cabbage and sauté for about 2 mins on medium heat or until the cabbage has softened. -Add in tomato sauce, salt and pepper to taste, then bring to a boil.
-Turn heat to medium-low then add remaining sausage and cook for about 10 mins or until cabbage is tender. -Serve over sliced Italian bread with desired toppings. Enjoy!

LUNCH: Buffalo Chicken Wrap with Salsa and Low Carb Tortilla Chips

Prep Time: 5 mins
Cook Time: 5 mins

Ingredients: 1 tbsp butter, 1/2 small onion, 3 oz buffalo chicken breast (grilled & chopped), 1/2 cup shredded lettuce, pinch of salt & pepper, 6 low carb tortilla chips.

Preparation:
-In a small bowl, mix butter and onions together, then microwave for about 30 secs. -To assemble, spread butter mixture over one side of each tortilla, then top with shredded lettuce, buffalo chicken and seasonings. -Roll up wrap then cut in half to serve. Garnish with an extra drizzle of buffalo sauce if desired. Enjoy!

DINNER: Paleo Meatloaf with Sweet Potato and Sage Casserole

Prep Time: 10 mins
Cook Time: 1 hour

Ingredients: 1/4 cup olive oil, 3 cloves garlic (minced), 2 cups ground beef or turkey, 2 cups low sodium organic tomato sauce, 2 sweet potatoes (peeled and chopped into cubes), 1/2 tsp dried oregano, salt & pepper to taste.

Preparation:

-In a large pot over medium-high heat, add oil then sauté garlic for about 30 secs. -Add in beef & seasonings to pot then stir well. -Cook for about 10 mins or until beef is cooked through. -Add in tomato sauce and sweet potato cubes, then turn heat to low, cover and cook for about 1 hour or until tender. Garnish with desired toppings. Enjoy!

DAY 64

BREAKFAST: Slow Cooker Beef Stew with mushrooms, cauliflower and red potatoes

Prep Time: 10 mins
Cook Time: 6 hours

Ingredients: 1lb beef stew meat (cut into chunks), 4 cloves garlic (minced), 1 cup uncooked red potatoes (cut into chunks), 2 cups cauliflower florets), 2 cups mushrooms (sliced), 3 cups canned diced tomatoes, 1 cup uncooked red beans, salt & pepper to taste.

Preparation:

-Season meat with salt and pepper to taste, then place in slow cooker. -Add remaining ingredients to slow cooker except for tomatoes and beans, stir well until well combined. Cover then cook on low heat for about 6-8 hours or until meat is tender. -In the last 30 mins of cooking, add in tomatoes and beans then cook for about 10 mins or until heated through. -Serve over desired veggies on sandwich or as desired. Enjoy!

LUNCH: Spicy Asian Tuna Caesar Salad with Cucumber & Tomato in a Pita Pocket

Prep Time: 5 mins
Cook Time: 15 mins

Ingredients: 6 cups romaine lettuce, 2 tbsp light mayo (low fat), 1 tbsp lime juice, 1/2 tsp sriracha, 1/2 cup sesame seeds, 4 slices canned tuna (packed in water), 28 slices cucumber, 4 large lettuce leaves.

Preparation:

-In a small bowl mix together light mayo and sriracha. -To assemble, place desired amount of lettuce in a bowl then top with tuna salad and cucumber. -Top with sesame seeds and serve in a pita pocket.

Enjoy!

DINNER: Paleo Lamb Burger (Serving size: 1 burger)

Prep Time: 10 mins
Cook Time: 8 mins

Ingredients: 1 lb. 93% lean ground lamb, 2 tbsp olive oil, 1/2 small onion (diced), salt & pepper to taste.

Preparation:
-In a large skillet over medium heat, add in oil then sauté diced onions until soft. -Add in lamb and season with salt and pepper to taste then cook until no longer pink. Remove from heat then set aside to cool. -Slice and serve on buns with desired toppings. Enjoy!

DAY 65

BREAKFAST: One-Pan Balsamic Shrimp Pasta with zucchini, asparagus and tomatoes

Prep Time: 5 mins
Cook Time: 25 mins

Ingredients: 1 lb. shrimp (peeled & deveined), 1 package angel hair pasta, 1/4 cup olive oil, 4 cloves garlic (minced), 4 cups zucchini (cubed), 1 cup asparagus (sliced), 2 cups tomatoes (sliced).

Preparation:
-In a large pan over medium heat, add oil then sauté garlic for 30 seconds. -Add in shrimp and cook for 2 mins per side or until pink. -Add in zucchini and cook for about 3 mins, add in asparagus and tomatoes, and cook for about 3-5 mins more. -In a small bowl, toss pasta with desired sauce and then serve over desired veggies. -Top with desired seasonings. Enjoy!

LUNCH: Tuna Salad Sandwich

Prep Time: 5 mins
Cook Time: 5 mins

Ingredients: 1 can tuna (packed in water), 1 tbsp low fat mayo, 1/2 cup celery (cut into sticks), 2 slices wheat or whole grain bread.

Preparation:

-In a small bowl mix tuna and mayo until combined. -To assemble, spread tuna salad on one slice of the bread and top with celery.   Cover with second slice of bread.   Enjoy! -Add desired toppings such as lettuce, tomato, onion and serve with a side of fruit if desired. Enjoy!

DINNER: Grilled Beef Fajitas and side of Guacamole over Romaine Lettuce and an Avocado Salsa

Prep Time: 1 hr. (Marinating the beef)
Cook Time: 15 mins

Ingredients: 1 lb. flank steak (sliced), 1 tbsp olive oil, 2 small onions (diced), 1 red pepper (sliced), 1 green pepper (sliced), salt & pepper to taste.

Preparation:

-Add beef to a medium bowl then add olive oil, garlic, onion, cilantro, salt & pepper to taste. Mix well then set aside. -In a large grill pan over medium-high heat, add in beef, then cook for 2-3 mins per side or until no longer pink. -Once cooked remove from heat and let rest for about 10 mins or just enough time for the juices to seep back into the meat. -To assemble, place desired amount of lettuce on plate and top with beef, tomatoes & onion then serve with guacamole and salsa. Enjoy!

DAY 66

BREAKFAST: Chopped Chicken Salad

Prep Time: 5 mins
Cook Time: 10 mins

Ingredients: 1 lb. chicken breast (diced), 2 tbsp olive oil, 1 small sweet onion (diced), 2 cloves garlic (minced), 2 cups broccoli florets, 1 cup carrots (sliced), 3 cup tomatoes, 3 tbsp lemon juice, 1/4 cup olive oil, salt & pepper to taste .

Preparation:

-In a medium bowl, add diced chicken, then lemon juice and season with salt & pepper to taste. Stir well until well combined. Set aside. -In a small skillet over medium heat, add in olive oil, then sauté onions until soft. Add in garlic and cook for 1 min then add in carrots and broccoli and cook for about 3-4 mins or until soft, stirring frequently. -Add to large bowl with chicken then stir well to combine.

-In a small bowl mix tomatoes and olive oil, season with salt & pepper to taste then spoon over the chicken mixture. Stir well again until combined then set aside to marinate for 10 mins or just enough time so the flavors can blend. -Serve over a bed of lettuce if desired and enjoy!

LUNCH: Grilled Salmon, Cucumber & Carrot Slaw in Pita Bread with Olive Oil Dressing

Prep Time: 10 mins
Cook Time: 15 mins

Ingredients: 16 oz salmon (cut into pieces), 1 tbsp olive oil, 4 cups thinly sliced cucumber, 2 cups finely shredded carrots, 1 small sweet onion (thinly sliced), 3 tbsp olive oil, 2 tbsp lemon juice, salt & pepper to taste.

Preparation:

-In a medium bowl add diced salmon then olive oil, then season with salt & pepper to taste and mix well until fish is well coated. Set aside for about 10 mins. -In a small bowl, whisk together lemon juice, onion, and olive oil, then season with salt & pepper to taste. -In a large grill pan over medium heat, add in sliced cucumber and carrots then sauté for 3-4 mins. Add in onion mixture and cook for another 2 mins then add in salmon, cook until no longer pink. -To assemble, slice pita bread and place lettuce on top then scoop salmon mixture onto lettuce and serve with olive oil dressing if desired. Enjoy!

DINNER: Chicken Panini with Caramelized Onions and Artichokes, served on a Roll with a Side Salad

Prep Time: 1 hr.
Cook Time: 20 mins

Ingredients: 2 lb. chicken breast (diced), 2 tbsp olive oil, 1 small sweet onion (diced), 1 red pepper (sliced), 1 green pepper (sliced), salt & pepper to taste.

Preparation:

-In a medium bowl, add diced chicken then olive oil, then season with salt & pepper to taste. Stir well until well combined. Set aside for about 10 mins. (Marinating the chicken)
-In a small skillet over medium heat, add in olive oil, then sauté onions until soft.   Add in garlic and cook for 1 min then add in peppers and cook for about 3-4 mins or until soft, stirring frequently. Preheat grill to medium heat. Lightly grease grill before placing chicken on it to prevent sticking.
-Cook chicken for about 7 mins per side or until no longer pink. Once cooked remove from heat and let rest for about 10 mins or just enough time for the juices to seep back into the meat.

-In a small bowl mix tomatoes and olive oil, season with salt & pepper to taste then spoon over the chicken mixture. Stir well again until combined then set aside to marinate for 10 mins or just enough time so the flavors can blend.
-Serve over a bed of lettuce if desired and enjoy!

DAY 67

BREAKFAST: Stroganoff

Prep Time: 4-5 mins
Cook Time: 10 mins

Ingredients: 1 lb. rib eye steak (sliced), 1 large onion (diced), 2 cloves garlic (minced), 2 tbsp olive oil, 2 tsp paprika, 1 cup mushrooms (diced), 2 to 3 cups baby spinach, 2 tbsp parmesan cheese, salt & pepper to taste.

Preparation:
-In a medium bowl add diced steak then onion & garlic and season with salt & pepper to taste then stir well until combined. Set aside for about 5 mins. -In a large skillet over medium heat, add in olive oil, then sauté mushrooms for 4-5 mins.   Add in spinach, onion and garlic and sauté for another 2-3 mins or until spinach is fully wilted. -Mix steak mixture with mushroom mixture then add cheese to the top of the steak. Stir well until well combined. Serve over a bed of spinach. -Enjoy!

LUNCH: Acorn Squash and Ham Sloppy Joes

Prep Time: 5 mins
Cook Time: 10 mins

Ingredients: 1 acorn squash (diced), ½ cup cherry tomatoes (diced), 1 green onion (sliced, chopped into 1 in pieces), 2 cloves garlic (chopped), 2 tsp olive oil, salt & pepper to taste.

Preparation:
-In a medium skillet over medium heat, add olive oil, then sauté onion for about 2-3 mins until soft, then add garlic and cook for another 1 min or until fragrant.
-Add in tomatoes, salt & pepper to taste, then cook for another 2 mins. Add in squash and cook for about 3-4 mins or until tender, stirring frequently.
-Mix together squash mixture with onion mixture then spoon into each of the buns. Top with ham slices and serve. Enjoy!

DINNER: **Paleo Philly Cheesesteak (vegan, low carb) with Cheesy Cauliflower & Broccoli or Roasted Brussels Sprouts**

Prep Time: 10 mins
Cook Time: 15 mins

Ingredients: 1 cup shiitake mushrooms (rehydrated until soft), 1 small sweet onion (sliced), 2 cloves garlic (minced), 2 tbsp olive oil, 4 leaves green cabbage (shredded), salt & pepper to taste.

Preparation:
-In a medium bowl, mix together mushrooms, onion and garlic then season with salt & pepper to taste. Add in olive oil and mix well.
-Sauté cabbage in olive oil over medium heat for 5 mins or until well wilted & tender, then add to large skillet over medium heat. Add in mushrooms mixture and cook for about 4-5 mins or until heated through. Serve over a bed of lettuce if desired. Enjoy!
-Enjoy!

DAY 68

BREAKFAST: **Lemon Chicken with asparagus, zucchini and mushrooms**

Prep Time: 10 mins
Cook Time: 10 mins

Ingredients: 2 skinless chicken breasts (diced), 4 cloves garlic (minced), salt & pepper to taste, 1 bunch asparagus (chopped into 1 in pieces), 2 small zucchini (sliced into half-moons) , mushroom, 3 small onions (halved and thinly sliced) , 2 tsp olive oil, juice from ½ of lemon.

Preparation:
-Add chicken to a large skillet over medium heat and cook until brown, then remove from pan and set aside. Reduce heat to low then add in olive oil.
-Add in onions, asparagus and garlic and season with salt & pepper to taste then sauté for about 5 mins. Add in lemon juice, cover and cook for another 2-3 mins or until soft. Stir well again until well combined, then set aside to cool slightly.
-Add zucchini, mushroom and season with salt & pepper to taste then sauté for about 3-4 mins until tender. Stir again until well combined, then set aside to cool slightly.
-Once vegetables have cooled slightly, stir together with chicken then serve. Enjoy!

LUNCH: **Caesar Salad**

Prep Time: 5 mins
Cook Time: 15 mins

Ingredients: 2 large romaine lettuce (washed, dried and chopped) , 1 cup cherry tomatoes (diced), 1 small red onion (thinly sliced), 2 cloves garlic (minced), 1 avocado (sliced into wedges) , 2 to 3 cups cooked chicken breast, 2 tbsp olive oil, juice from ½ of lemon.

Preparation:

-In a medium bowl, stir together lettuce and tomatoes, then season with salt & pepper to taste, then set aside.
Add in olive oil, garlic and lemon juice, stirring constantly until well combined. Set aside for 10 mins or so.
-Once ready top salad with avocado and chicken then serve. Enjoy!

DINNER: **Chicken Chorizo Patties with Cauliflower Mash & Guacamole**

Prep Time: 10 mins
Cook Time: 35 mins

Ingredients: 2 chicken breasts (diced), salt & pepper to taste, 1 can chickpeas (drained and rinsed), 1 clove garlic (minced), 1 large onion (sliced into rings), 2 tsp olive oil, crushed tomatoes, 2 tsp paprika, ½ cup green onions, salt & pepper to taste.

Preparation:

-Add chicken to a large mixing bowl and season with salt & pepper to taste then stir well until well combined. Add in chickpeas, garlic, onion, and tomato paste then mix well making sure everything is mixed together well. Season with paprika to taste then set aside for 10 mins or so.
-Add in green onions and mix again until everything is well combined. Season with salt & pepper to taste then set aside for an hour or so (3x this would be better).
-Once ready add in cauliflower and mix well until everything is evenly distributed throughout the cauliflower mash. Set aside while the patties are cooking.
-To cook the patties, add olive oil to a large skillet over medium heat, then spoon mixture into skillet in balls. Cook each side for about 2-3 mins or until golden brown then serve. Enjoy!

DAY 69

BREAKFAST: Meatball Parmesan Soup

Prep Time: 10 mins
Cook Time: 20 mins

Ingredients: 1 lb. ground beef (or turkey), 1 cup carrots (shredded), 2 tsp olive oil, 1/2 onion (diced), 2 cloves garlic (minced), 1 tsp oregano, 1 can diced tomatoes (undrained) , 4 cups tomato sauce, chicken stock (1 cup liquid, 4 cups water).

Preparation:

-Add ground beef to a large saucepan over medium heat and cook until browned then add in oregano and stir. Add in onion and garlic and cook until onions are soft. Add in tomatoes and tomato sauce and stir. Reduce heat to low, then add in chicken stock, then cover and simmer for about 15 mins or until meat is cooked through. Stir well often. -Add carrot shreds, season with oregano, salt & pepper to taste and mix until well combined then set aside for 10 mins or so.
-Remove from heat. -Serve soup over a bed of lettuce if desired, then top with meatballs and serve.
-Enjoy!

LUNCH: Baked Tilapia & Broccoli (vegan, low carb)

Prep Time: 15 mins
Cook Time: 25 mins

Ingredients: 2 tilapia fillets (boneless and skinless), 1 head broccoli (or any greens of choice), olive oil, salt & pepper to taste.

Preparation:
-Preheat oven to 180c. Line a baking sheet with tin foil and set aside. Add fillets to a large mixing bowl and season with salt, pepper and olive oil then toss well until well coated. Set aside for about 10 mins or so until fish is completely cooked through.
-Meanwhile, add broccoli to a medium-sized pot over medium heat and cook for about 2 mins until the broccoli begins to soften. Season with salt & pepper to taste then set aside for about 15 mins or so. -If broccoli still seems a little hard after 15 mins, add a splash of water then cover and cook for another few mins. Set aside to cool slightly.
-Once ready, spoon broccoli onto a separate plate and top with fillets then serve. Enjoy!

DINNER: Paleo Chicken Pot Pie, served with a Side Salad with Toasted Almonds and Lemon Basil Oil

Prep Time: 10 mins
Cook Time: 45 mins

Ingredients: 3 chicken breasts (diced), 1 cup baby carrots (halved lengthwise), 2 small onions (sliced into strips), 1/2 cup green peas, 1 tbsp olive oil, salt & pepper to taste.

Preparation:

-Add chicken to a large mixing bowl and season with salt & pepper to taste then stir well until well combined. Add in carrots, onion, and peas then mix again until everything is well combined. Set aside for about 15 mins or so. -Cut pastry into 5-inch squares placing on a baking sheet lined with parchment paper and spread 1 tbsp olive oil over the tops of each square. Bake for about 15 mins at 400F, turn off heat and leave in oven for another 20 mins or until golden brown in color. Remove from oven set aside to cool slightly. -Once ready, spoon chicken mixture onto each square, then top with another square. Serve with a side salad. Enjoy!

DAY 70

BREAKFAST: Southwest Turkey Burgers with Lime Avocado Slaw

Prep Time: 15 mins
Cook Time: 30 mins

Ingredients: 1 lb. ground turkey, 1 tsp cumin, 1 tsp chili powder or to taste, salt & pepper to taste, 1/2 cup onion (diced), 2 cloves garlic (minced), ½ jalapeno (diced), 2 tbsp lime juice, salsa of choice.

Preparation:

-Add ground turkey to a large mixing bowl and season with cumin, chili powder, salt & pepper to taste, then stir well until well combined. Add minced garlic and diced jalapeño and stir until everything is well combined. Set aside for 10 mins or so.
-In the meantime, heat a large skillet over medium heat, add half of the onion, and cook until browned. Once cooked remove from pan and set aside. Add in the rest of the onion to the same pan and sauté for about 2 mins then set aside to cool slightly.
-Once ready add lime juice, salsa, cooked onions and garlic to the bowl containing the turkey mixture then mix well until everything is evenly distributed.

-Add oil to a medium-sized skillet over medium heat, then spoon mixture into skillet in balls. Cook each side for about 2-3 mins or until golden brown then serve with lime avocado slaw on top if desired. Enjoy!

LUNCH: **Greek Chicken Salad**

Prep Time: 10 mins
Cook Time: 15 mins

Ingredients: 1 lb. of chicken breast (diced), fresh spinach leaves, fresh lemon juice to taste, salt & pepper to taste, 1-2 cloves garlic (minced).

Preparation:
-Add chicken to a large mixing bowl then season with salt & pepper to taste. Add in garlic and stir well until everything is evenly distributed. Set aside for about 20 mins or so then grill on BBQ rack over medium heat. Cook for about 15 mins or until chicken is cooked through. Cover grill and cook for about another 5 mins or until cooked through. Serve with lemon spinach salad on top.
-Enjoy!

DINNER: **Paleo Cauliflower & Leek Soup with Crumbled Bacon on top with a piece of Whole Wheat Toasted Bread**

Prep Time: 5 mins
Cook Time: 20 mins
Ingredients: 1-2 florets of cauliflower, 1 tbsp olive oil, sea salt and pepper to taste, 1 onion (diced), 2 cloves garlic (minced).

Preparation:
-Add cauliflower to a large mixing bowl. Add in olive oil and sea salt & pepper to taste, then toss well until well combined. Add in diced onion and minced garlic then stir once again until everything is evenly distributed. Set aside for about 15 mins or so.
-Heat oven to 200F (fan). Line a baking sheet with tin foil and spray the tin foil with non-stick cooking spray then place cauliflower florets on a baking sheet and bake for about 15 mins or until cooked through but still firm to the touch. Serve with bread if desired. Enjoy!

DAY 71

BREAKFAST: **Bacon, Egg & Cheese Breakfast Sandwich on English Muffin**

Prep Time: 15 mins
Cook Time: 20 mins

Ingredients: 6 slices bacon (cooked), 2 slices of whole wheat or grain-free bread, 1-2 tsp garlic powder, ½ cup cheddar cheese (shredded), 1 egg (scrambled), salt & pepper to taste.

Preparation:
-Spread 1 tsp of garlic powder over the outside slices of bread then place in a medium-sized skillet. Cook each side for about 1-2 mins or until golden brown and toasted. Set aside to cool slightly. -Once ready, spread ½ cup cheese over the untoasted sides of each slice of bread then layer with egg and bacon on one slice followed by another layer of cheese. Top with the other slice of bread and serve with a side of fruit if desired. Enjoy!

LUNCH: **Chicken Parmesan Pasta Bake with Spinach and Peppers**

Prep Time: 5 mins
Cook Time: 30 mins

Ingredients: 1 lb. chicken breast (diced), 1 cup spinach, ¼ red bell pepper (diced), ½ yellow bell pepper (diced), 1 tbsp olive oil, salt & pepper to taste, 2 cloves garlic (minced).

Preparation:
-Add chicken to a medium-sized mixing bowl, then season with salt & pepper. Add in all other ingredients then stir well until everything is evenly distributed. Set aside for 20 mins or so then bake covered at 350F for about 15 mins or until chicken is cooked through and tender. Serve with pasta and veggies of choice if desired.

DINNER: **Shrimp Scampi Stir-fry over Brown Rice Pasta or Quinoa Pilaf**

Prep Time: 15 mins
Cook Time: 30 mins

Ingredients: 2 lbs. shrimp (peeled and deveined), 1 tbsp olive oil, 1 tsp garlic salt, 1 tsp onion powder, ½ cup crushed tomatoes (crushed), 1 cup quinoa (washed well), 1 cup of chicken broth or stock.

Preparation:

-Add olive oil to a large skillet over medium heat then add in shrimp and cook for about 3 mins or until shrimp is pink. Add in garlic salt & onion powder and stir well until evenly distributed. Add crushed tomatoes and stir again until evenly distributed. Cook for about 5 mins then add in quinoa and chicken broth/stock. Stir well, then cover pan with lid and reduce heat to low. Cook for about 20 mins or until liquid is absorbed completely, stirring occasionally during the cooking process. Serve with a side of rice or quinoa if desired. Enjoy!

DAY 72

BREAKFAST: **Chicken Sausage Zucchini Noodle Soup with cherry tomatoes, peppers and spinach**

Prep Time: 5 mins
Cook Time: 20 mins

Ingredients: 1 lb. chicken breast (diced), 1 small onion (diced),. 4 large zucchini (sliced into noodle-like strips), 1 cup cherry tomatoes (halved), ½ yellow bell pepper (diced), ½ red bell pepper (diced), 2 cups of spinach, 2 cups of chicken broth/stock, salt & pepper to taste.

Preparation:

-Add stock and diced onion to a large mixing bowl. Add in chicken and stir well until evenly distributed, then add in tomatoes, peppers and zucchini noodles. Cook for about 20 mins covered or until zucchini is cooked through but still firm to the touch.
Serve with tortilla chips if desired. Enjoy!

LUNCH: **Cheezy Chicken Veggie Soup with Cucumber and Garlic Rye Crackers**

Prep Time: 15 mins
Cook Time: 20 mins
Ingredients: 1 cup cherry tomatoes (halved), 1 cup zucchini (sliced into noodle-like strips), 1 yellow onion (chopped), 2 cloves garlic (minced), 2 tbsp olive oil, 2 cups chicken breast (diced or cut into small chunks), ¾ cup cheddar cheese (shredded), ½ cup cream cheese, salt & pepper to taste.

Preparation:

-Sautee garlic and onions in olive oil over medium heat until onions are translucent.   Add in all other veggies, then stir well again until evenly coated with olive oil. Turn heat off, then add in chicken & cheeses and stir until cheese is melted. Stir in cherry tomatoes & zucchini noodles.
Cover pan with lid and cook for about 20 mins or until zucchini is cooked through but still tender to the touch. Serve with garlic rye crackers if desired. Enjoy!

DINNER: Grilled Chicken & Asparagus Stir-fry with Zucchini, Mango and Orange Salsa on a Bed of Greens
Prep Time: 15 mins
Cook Time: 15 mins

Ingredients: 2 lbs chicken breast (cut into large chunks), ½ cup orange segments (diced), 1 cup asparagus (cut into small bite-sized pieces), ¼ red onion (finely chopped or diced), 2 cups red leaf lettuce or spinach, 1 tbsp olive oil, salt & pepper to taste.

Preparation:
-Add oil to a large skillet over medium heat then add in onions and cook for about 1 min or until fragrant.
Add in chicken and stir it around for about 2 mins or until chicken is pink on the outside.
Add in asparagus and orange segments then stir well again until evenly distributed. Cover pan with lid and let it cook for about 10 mins or until asparagus is tender but still has a slight crunch, stirring occasionally during the cooking process. Season with salt & pepper to taste if desired. Serve over lettuce or spinach with a side of bread if desired. Enjoy!

DAY 73

BREAKFAST: Spicy Shrimp Skewers with Avocado Mango Salsa
Prep Time: 10 mins
Cook Time: 15 mins

Ingredients: 2 cups of shrimp (peeled and deveined), 1 tbsp olive oil, 2 tsp chipotle powder, salt &. pepper to taste, ½ cup of mango (diced), ½ cup avocado (diced), ¼ red onion (finely diced or thinly sliced), 1 tbsp fresh lime juice, 1 tbsp cilantro (chopped), 8 grape tomatoes

Preparation:
-Stir. together lime juice, oil, chipotle powder and salt & pepper.

Toss shrimp with this mixture then thread each piece on a wooden skewer. Grill skewers over medium heat for about 5 mins or until shrimp is pink on the outside and no longer translucent. Remove skewers from grill and set aside. Add in all other ingredients to a medium mixing bowl, then stir well until smooth and evenly distributed. Serve with tortilla chips if desired. Enjoy!

LUNCH: **Turkey Burgers with Avocado Salsa, Romaine Lettuce and Low Carb Tortilla Chips**

Prep Time: 15 mins
Cook Time: 15 mins

Ingredients: 1 lb. ground turkey (extra lean), ½ cup shredded cabbage or lettuce, ½ of an avocado (diced), 1 tbsp cilantro (chopped), 1 tbsp cumin powder, salt & pepper to taste.

Preparation:
-Mix all ingredients in a large mixing bowl, then bring the mixture together with your hands. Form into patties and place on the grill over medium heat. Place burgers on the grill, then cover the grill and cook for about 15 mins or until turkey is fully cooked through but still has a slight pinkness to it. Serve with romaine lettuce, salsa, and low carb tortilla chips if desired. Enjoy!

DINNER: **Paleo Meatloaf (vegan, low carb) with Sweet Potatoes and Pecans**

Prep Time: 15 mins
Cook Time: 45 mins

Ingredients: 3 small sweet potatoes (peeled & cut into small cubes), 1 cup of onion (diced), 2 lbs. ground beef (extra lean), 2 large eggs, 1 cup coconut milk, 2 tbsp garlic powder, 1 tbsp salt & pepper to taste.

Preparation:
-Preheat oven to 375 degrees. Add all ingredients to a large mixing bowl, then mix with your hands or a wooden spoon until well combined, smashing the sweet potatoes into the ground beef. Press mixture into a baking pan that has been sprayed with non-stick spray, then bake in preheated oven for about 45 mins or until meat is cooked through and no longer pink in the center. Cut into 6 slices and serve with a side of sweet potatoes and pecans if desired. Enjoy!

DAY 74

BREAKFAST: Asian Shrimp Noodle Bowl with Veggies and Ginger Soy Sauce

Prep Time: 15 mins
Cook Time: 20 mins

Ingredients: 1 cup shrimp (peeled & deveined), 1 tbsp olive oil, 1 cup asparagus (topped and tailed then cut into 2-inch pieces), 2 cups shiitake mushrooms (sliced or diced), ½ cup carrots (grated or sliced), ½ red pepper (sliced), ½ yellow pepper(sliced), ½ cup bamboo shoots, 2 cloves garlic (minced), 1 tsp ginger powder, salt & pepper to taste.

Preparation:
-Bring a large pot of water to a boil over high heat then add in shrimp and cook for 6 minutes or until shrimp is opaque in color (cooking time will depend on your size of shrimp). Drain the water off and set it aside. Add oil to a large skillet over medium heat, then add in all other veggies & spices then stir well until evenly coated with olive oil. Add cooked shrimp back into the sauce & stir well again until all pieces are evenly distributed. Simmer over low heat for about 20 mins or until carrots are tender but still have a slight crunch. Season with salt and pepper to taste if desired. Serve with cooked rice noodles, veggies and ginger soy sauce if desired. Enjoy!

LUNCH: Shrimp Scampi Pasta Bake with Spinach and Parmesan

Prep Time: 20 mins
Cook Time: 20 mins

Ingredients: 1 lb of gluten-free pasta (your choice), 1 lb shrimp (peeled & deveined), 2 cups spinach (de-stemmed & blanched for about 5 minutes or until tender then chopped), 1 cup mushrooms, ½ red onion (thinly sliced), 3 cloves of garlic (minced), olive oil for drizzling.

Preparation:
-Bring a large pot of water to a boil over high heat, add pasta, and cook according to package directions. While pasta is cooking, bring a large skillet with olive oil to medium heat, then add in shrimp, spinach, onions and garlic. Cook shrimp till they turn pink on the outside but are still slightly translucent in color. Add cooked pasta into the pan with the other ingredients then stir well until evenly distributed. Drizzle with olive oil as desired & serve warm. Enjoy!

DINNER: **Paleo Roasted Red Chili (vegan, gluten free)**

Prep Time: 5 mins

Ingredients: 1 red bell pepper (chopped), ½ cup onion (chopped), 2 plum tomatoes (quartered), 1 tbsp olive oil, 2 cloves of garlic (minced), 1 tsp oregano, ¼ tsp cumin powder, salt & pepper to taste.

Preparation:

-Remove seeds from the red pepper, then dice. Add oil to a large skillet over medium heat, add in the red pepper, onion & spices, then stir well until veggies are coated well. Cook for about 5 mins or until veggies have softened but not browned. Add in tomatoes and cook for about 5 mins more on low heat. Serve warm with rice if desired or enjoy alone.

DAY 75

BREAKFAST: **Grilled Cheese with Ham and Tomato**

Prep Time: 10 mins
Cook Time: 10 mins

Ingredients: 2 slices of white bread or gluten free bread, 1 piece of ham (sliced), 1 large tomato, 1 slice of cheddar cheese (optional).

Preparation:

-Take white bread or gluten free bread and lay it out on a flat surface. Place ham, tomato and cheese on top of one piece of bread, then place other piece of bread over the top and press down to secure in place. Grill over medium heat until cheese melts (about 2 mins), then flip and grill on the other side. Serve warm with your choice of side.

-Enjoy!

LUNCH: **Spicy Buffalo Chicken with Pesto in a Pita Pocket**

Prep Time: 10 mins
Cook Time: 15 mins

Ingredients: 1 chicken breast (sliced into strips), ½ cup mozzarella cheese (shredded), 1 tbsp. buffalo sauce, 2 tsp pesto, 1 pita pocket (cut in half).

Preparation:

-Place chicken strips into a large bowl then add buffalo sauce and pesto. Stir well until chicken is completely coated with the mixture. Cook chicken in a large skillet over medium heat for about 7-10 mins or until cooked through and no longer pink in the center. Add mozzarella cheese, stir well then remove from heat. Stuff pita pocket with spicy buffalo chicken then drizzle with low carb pizza sauce if desired. Enjoy!

DINNER: Bacon Wrapped Chicken Breasts Over Spicy Kale Chips

Prep Time: 10 mins
Cook Time: 15 mins

Ingredients: 2 chicken breast (sliced into strips), 1 cup spinach leaves, 1 tbsp. olive oil, ½ tsp garlic powder, ¼ tsp paprika.

Preparation:
-In a large bowl, add in chicken strips and spices then fold in spinach leaves. Place chicken on a large baking sheet with sides, then drizzle with olive oil and toss until evenly coated. Bake at 350 degrees for about 15 mins or until cooked through.
-While chicken is cooking in the oven, place kale leaves in a medium skillet over medium heat, then drizzle with olive oil and toss until kale is evenly coated. Sauté for about 2-3 mins or until leaves are slightly wilted. Serve warm with bacon wrapped chicken. Enjoy!

DAY 76

BREAKFAST: Scrambled Egg Wrap

Prep Time: 10 mins
Cook Time: 5 mins

Ingredients: 2 large eggs (scrambled), 1 tsp coconut oil, ½ cup spinach, ½ cup red pepper, 2 tbsp sliced jalapeños, salt & pepper to taste.

Preparation:
-Take 2 large eggs and scramble them in the coconut oil over medium heat for about 2 mins or until cooked through. Add in all other ingredients & season with salt & pepper to your desired taste then stir well. Serve warm with tortilla wrap and enjoy!
-Enjoy!

LUNCH: Meatball Subs with Melted Mozzarella and Tomato Sauce on Garlic Toast Points

Prep Time: 15 mins
Cook Time: 20 mins

Ingredients: 6 cooked & slightly cooled meatballs, ¼ cup marinara sauce, 6 slices of gluten free bread or your choice of bread (sliced), 1 cup mozzarella cheese (shredded), garlic powder, salt & pepper to taste.

Preparation:
-Lay out each slice of bread and spread with 2 tbsp marinara sauce then add 2 slices of cheese. Take a slice of toast, flatten slightly and place a meatball on top. Wrap sandwich by folding in sides and tucking the top under the bottom. Repeat this process for all sandwiches. Cook in a large skillet over medium heat for about 5 mins or until tops are slightly toasted & cheese is melted.
-Enjoy!

DINNER: Paleo Chicken & Vegetable Soup with Zucchini Noodles

Prep Time: 15 mins
Cook Time: 20 mins

Ingredients: 2 chicken breasts (sliced into strips), 1 red onion (diced), ½ cup celery, 1 clove of garlic (cloves minced), 5 cups chicken broth, ½ tsp oregano, ¼ tsp thyme, half an avocado (diced).

Preparation:
-In a large bowl add in chicken and toss to coat with olive oil then season with oregano, thyme, and salt & pepper to your desired taste. Add onion and celery, then cook over medium heat for about 6-8 mins or until the chicken is no longer pink in the center. Add in garlic, broth and half an avocado then bring mixture to a boil. Reduce heat to low & simmer for about 15 mins or until veggies are tender. Serve warm with zucchini noodles.

DAY 77

BREAKFAST: Buffalo Chicken Salad with celery, carrots, chickpeas and Ranch dressing

Prep Time: 10 mins

Ingredients: 1 chicken breast (sliced into strips), ¼ cup buffalo sauce, ½ cup celery, ½ cup carrots, ¼ cup chickpeas (cooked), 2 tbsp. grated cheddar cheese (optional), ½ tsp ranch dressing.

Preparation:
-In a large bowl add in chicken then toss to coat with buffalo sauce. Place chicken on a large baking sheet with sides, drizzle with ranch dressing if desired & toss to coat. Bake at 350 degrees for about 10 mins or until cooked through & no longer pink in the center. Remove from oven & let cool then add all other ingredients and toss to combine. Serve cold or at room temperature. Enjoy!
-Enjoy!

LUNCH: Grilled Cheese Sandwich on Cheddar, Tomato Basil Bread with Raspberries

Prep Time: 10 mins
Cook Time: 15 mins

Ingredients: 2 slices of cheddar, tomato basil bread, 1 tbsp. butter, ½ cup raspberries (fresh or frozen is fine), pinch salt & pepper to taste.

Preparation:
-Butter both sides of bread, then place in a large skillet over medium heat. Place cheese on one slice of bread and tomato basil bread on the other slice. Toast both sides of bread before flipping, then continue to cook until cheese is melted. Remove from heat and top with salt & pepper. Cut in half and top with raspberries. Enjoy!

DINNER: Paleo Turkey Chili (vegan, low carb) with Toasted Pumpkin Seeds

Prep Time: 15 mins
Cook Time: 20 mins

Ingredients: 1 lb. ground turkey (browned), 2 cans of beans, 3 cups beef broth, 1 red pepper (diced), 1 tsp cumin powder, ¼ tsp oregano, 1 tbsp chili powder, ½ tsp garlic powder.

Preparation:

-In a large skillet over medium heat add in Turkey and cook until it is no longer pink in the center. Remove from heat & set aside. In a large pot, add in beans & broth, then add in raw diced pepper & spices. Bring mixture to a boil, then reduce heat to low and simmer uncovered for about 10 mins or until veggies are tender. Add cooked turkey to pot, then serve warm with toasted pumpkin seeds.

DAY 78

BREAKFAST: Greek Tuna Pita Sandwich

Prep Time: 5 mins
Cook Time: 0 mins

Ingredients: 1 bowl of spinach (cooked), 2 pita breads, 1 tsp olive oil, 2 tbsp chopped cucumber, 1 can of tuna in water (drained), lemon juice to taste.

Preparation:

-In a large bowl, add spinach, then squeeze lemon juice in & toss to coat. Add in tuna & cucumber then drizzle with olive oil. Divide mixture into each pita bread then serve.

LUNCH: Broccoli, Carrot & Cheddar Soup with Cilantro Croutons

Prep Time: 10 mins
Cook Time: 10 mins

Ingredients: 1 medium head of broccoli (chopped into small florets), ½ cup shredded carrots (sliced), 2 cloves of garlic (diced), 2 tbsp fresh cilantro leaves (chopped), 2 green onions (sliced).

Preparation:

-In a large pot add in broccoli then cover with water. Bring to a boil, then reduce heat to low and cook for about 7 mins or until broccoli is tender. Strain broccoli then set aside. Add in carrots & garlic to the same pot, bring all ingredients to a simmer, cover, and cook for another 6-8 minutes or until carrot is tender. Remove from heat and add in cooked broccoli, cilantro and green onions then blend mixture with a hand blender until smooth. Top with croutons and serve warm.

DINNER: Cauliflower Mash & Roasted Broccoli or Eggplant Puree (vegan, low carb)

Prep Time: 10 mins
Cook Time: 20 mins

Ingredients: Cauliflower (2 heads), broccoli (1 head), eggplant (1 medium).

Preparation:

-Cut cauliflower in small florets, then place in a large pot with some water. Boil over medium heat for about 10-15 mins or until cauliflower is tender. Strain cauliflower then place back into same pot and add in broccoli, cover, and cook for an additional 5-8 mins or until broccoli is tender. Remove from heat & set aside. In a large covered skillet over medium heat, roast eggplant until it is tender. Remove from heat and set aside. In a large skillet over medium heat roast broccoli until it is tender. Remove from heat & set aside. Place the cauliflower into a large mixing bowl then add eggplant, broccoli and any other ingredients you wish to add (such as fresh herbs). Blend with a hand blender until smooth. Serve warm or at room temperature.

DAY 79

BREAKFAST: Hearty Beef Soup with quinoa, potatoes and kale

Prep Time: 30 mins
Cook Time: 45 mins

Ingredients: 1 lb. ground beef (browned), 2 onions (diced), 3 stalks of celery (diced), 1 tbsp. olive oil, 4 cloves of garlic (crushed), 1 can of diced green chiles (drained).

Preparation:

-Peel the potatoes, then chop into small chunks. Place in a large stockpot & cover with water then boil for about 15 mins or until fork tender. Add in browned ground beef to pot then mash with potato chunks once cooked. Add in remaining ingredients, then simmer for about 30 mins or until celery is tender. Serve warm topped with cheese or sour cream if desired.

Preparation:

-In a medium size mixing bowl whisk 3 eggs, 1 tbsp. olive oil, salt & pepper. Add in ½ cup shredded cheddar cheese to the bowl then fold egg mixture into the cheddar cheese until it is fully combined. In a large skillet, add in butter or oil over medium heat, then pour egg mixture into pan. Cook for about 2 mins on each side or until golden brown. Remove from heat & set aside for later use in lunch meal.

LUNCH: **Vegetable Omelet**

Prep Time: 5 mins
Cook Time: 12-15 mins

Ingredients: 1/2 cup chopped tomatoes, 8 egg whites, 1 tbsp fresh parsley (chopped), 2 tbsp water, 1 tsp olive oil, 1 cup of spinach (fresh or frozen), chopped broccoli, salt & pepper to taste.

Preparation:

-In a large mixing bowl whisk egg whites then add in salt & pepper to taste. In a medium-sized skillet over medium heat add in olive oil then add in chopped tomatoes. Let cook until tomatoes have softened, then add in fresh chopped parsley then cook for another 30 seconds. In a separate large skillet over medium heat melt 2 tbsp butter, 1 tbsp olive oil and eggs. Add egg mixture to pan, cook for about 2-3 mins on each side or until golden brown and cooked through (to prevent curling you may want to flip the omelet sooner). Place next to spinach & broccoli on a plate with cheese if desired.

DINNER: **Beef Stew & Cauliflower Mash (vegan, low carb)**

Prep Time: 20 mins
Cook Time: 1 hr. 15 mins

Ingredients: 1 lb. stew meat (browned) 3 cloves of garlic (chopped), salt & pepper to taste, 2 cups of water, chopped carrots & celery, 1 can of diced tomatoes (undrained), 2 tbsp tomato paste.

Preparation:

-Peel the potato then chop into small chunks. Place in a large pot and cover with water then boil for about 10-15 mins or until fork tender. Drain & set aside for later use. Add olive oil over medium heat in a large stockpot or Dutch oven, then brown ground beef (drain fat). Add in garlic, salt & pepper, then cook for another 2 mins until garlic is fragrant. Add in carrots & celery, then season with salt & pepper to taste. Stir in chopped tomatoes, then add in diced potatoes and broth (about 1 cup of water) to the stockpot. Bring all ingredients to a simmer then cook for about 45-60 mins or until stew meat is tender. Once finished serve over cauliflower mash.

DAY 80

BREAKFAST: Fish Tacos in Corn Tortillas with Tomatillo Salsa (vegan, low carb)

Prep Time: 15 mins
Cook Time: 15 mins

Ingredients: 1 lb. tilapia fillets, 1 cup of rinsed black beans, 2 cups. of fresh corn kernels, 1 tbsp. olive oil, 2 cloves of garlic (crushed), 1 can chopped green chiles (drained).

Preparation:
-In a medium-sized mixing bowl whisk eggs then add in salt & pepper to taste. In a large skillet over medium heat, add olive oil, fish fillets, and cook for about 5 mins on each side or until browned. Add in black beans, tomatoes and green chiles, then stir well. Pull out the pan off heat & pour egg mixture into skillet. Stir together well & continue cooking until egg is almost cooked through (to prevent curling you may want to flip the omelet sooner). Serve warm in corn tortillas.

LUNCH: Spicy Shrimp Tacos in Corn Tortillas with Lime Sour Cream Sauce & Avocado Salsa (vegan, low carb)

Prep Time: 15 mins
Cook Time: 5 mins

Ingredients: 8 medium shrimp, 2 tbsp lime juice, 1 clove garlic (minced), 1/4 tsp. cumin, 1/4 tsp. chili powder, 1 tsp olive oil, salt & pepper to taste.

Preparation:
-In a large skillet over medium-high heat, add olive oil and shrimp. Brown for about 2 mins on each side or until browned and cooked through. In a small bowl whisk together lime juice, garlic, cumin, salt & pepper to taste, then pour over shrimp. Stir well & once shrimp is cooked through, remove from heat. Lay 3-4 equal sized shrimp on each corn tortilla with your choice of toppings.
 -In a medium-sized mixing bowl whisk sour cream, lime juice, salt & pepper to taste. Serve with avocado & shrimp tacos.

DINNER: Chicken Fried Cauliflower Tots with a Side Salad and Zucchini Fries (vegan, low carb)

Prep Time: 15 mins

Cook Time: 20 mins

Ingredients: 1 pound of cauliflower (cut into florets), 2 eggs, 1 cup flour (all-purpose), 3 tsp. salt, 1 tsp. pepper, olive oil to coat bottom of skillet, zucchini fritters.

Preparation:
-In a large skillet over medium heat, add olive oil and cut cauliflower florets. Toss to coat in oil, then season with salt & pepper to taste. Turn heat down low & cook for about 5 mins on each side or until tender and slightly browned on edges. In a separate bowl combine eggs, flour, salt & pepper to taste. Coat cauliflower mixture in egg mixture then fry for about 1-2 mins on each side or until golden brown and cooked through. Drain excess oil from skillet, then top with zucchini fritters. Serve warm with side salad & ranch dressing.

DAY 81

BREAKFAST: **Vegetarian Lasagna with Mushrooms & Spinach (vegan, low carb)**

Prep Time: 15 mins
Cook Time: 35 mins

Ingredients: 2 tbsp olive oil, 1 onion (chopped), 3 cloves garlic (minced), 1-pound mushrooms (sliced), 10 oz baby spinach leaves, 1 jar (24 oz) marinara sauce, 12 lasagna noodles, 15 oz ricotta cheese, 1 egg, 2 tbsp parsley (chopped), 1/2 cup Parmesan cheese (grated), salt & pepper to taste.

Preparation:
-In a large pot of boiling water, cook lasagna noodles according to package instructions. In a separate skillet over medium heat, add olive oil, then add onions, garlic & mushrooms. Sauté for about 5 mins or until tender then season with salt & pepper to taste. Stir in spinach leaves & cook for 1-2 mins or until wilted. Once noodles are cooked, drain water, then rinse with cold water. In a large baking dish, spread 1/2 cup of marinara sauce evenly on the bottom then top with 6 noodles. Spread ricotta cheese mixture over noodles, then top with mushroom & spinach mixture. Repeat layers ending with noodles & sauce. Cover with foil then bake for about 30 minutes or until heated through. Remove from oven then let cool for 5 mins before serving.

LUNCH: **Thin Crust Chicken Pizza with Arugula and Parmesan Cheese (vegan, low carb)**

Prep Time: 15 mins
Cook Time: 10 mins

Ingredients: 1/2-pound chicken breast (sliced), 1/4 cup tomato sauce, 1/4 cup mozzarella cheese (shredded), 1 tbsp Parmesan cheese (grated), 2 cloves garlic (minced), 1/4 tsp. oregano, 1/4 tsp. basil, salt & pepper to taste, 1/2 cup arugula leaves.

Preparation:
-In a small bowl, whisk together tomato sauce, garlic, oregano, basil, salt & pepper to taste. Set aside. Preheat oven to 350 degrees F (175 degrees C). Over medium-high heat, cook chicken until browned and cooked through in a large skillet. Remove from heat then chop into bite-sized pieces. In a small bowl, mix together mozzarella cheese & Parmesan cheese. On a large baking sheet, spread 1/4 cup of tomato sauce mixture evenly then top with chicken pieces. Sprinkle shredded cheese over chicken then bake for about 10 mins or until cheese is melted and bubbly. Remove from oven then top with arugula leaves. Serve warm.

DINNER: **Paleo Nachos with Spicy Sour Cream, Avocado & Pico de Gallo (vegan, low carb)**

Prep Time: 10 mins
Cook Time: 5 mins

Ingredients: 1/2 head cauliflower (riced), 1/4 cup almond flour, 1 tsp. chili powder, 1/2 tsp. cumin, salt & pepper to taste, olive oil, 2 avocados (sliced), 1/4 cup sour cream, 1/4 cup Pico de Gallo.

Preparation:
-In a large bowl, mix riced cauliflower, almond flour, chili powder, cumin, salt & pepper to taste. Heat olive oil in a large skillet over medium-high heat then add cauliflower mixture. Stir fry for about 5 mins or until tender. Remove from heat, then top with avocado slices, sour cream & Pico de Gallo. Serve warm.

DAY 82

BREAKFAST: Stir-Fry Pork Rice Bowl (low carb)

Prep Time: 10 mins
Cook Time: 10 mins

Ingredients: 1/4-pound pork tenderloin (sliced), 1/4 cup soy sauce, 1 tbsp rice vinegar, 1 tbsp honey, 1 clove garlic (minced), 1/4 tsp, ginger powder, salt & pepper to taste, 2 tbsp olive oil, 1 head broccoli (chopped), 1 red pepper (sliced), 1/2 cup brown rice.

Preparation:
-In a small bowl whisk together soy sauce, rice vinegar, honey, garlic & ginger powder. Set aside. Season pork slices with salt & pepper to taste. Heat olive oil in a large skillet over medium-high heat then add pork. Cook for about 3-5 minutes per side or until browned. Remove from heat then add broccoli & red pepper to the same skillet. Stir fry for about 3-5 mins or until tender. Add soy sauce mixture to the pan & cook for 1 minute or until heated through. Serve over brown rice.

LUNCH: Turkey Reuben Sandwiches (with sauerkraut)

Prep Time: 10 mins
Cook Time: 10 mins

Ingredients: 4 slices rye bread, 1/4 cup mayonnaise, 1 tbsp yellow mustard, 8 oz turkey breast (sliced), 1/4 cup sauerkraut, 1/4 cup Swiss cheese (shredded), 1 tbsp butter.

Preparation:
-In a small bowl mix together mayonnaise & mustard. Spread mixture on one side of each slice of bread then top 2 slices with turkey, sauerkraut, Swiss cheese & remaining bread slices. Heat butter in a large skillet over medium heat. Place sandwiches in the skillet then cook for about 3-5 minutes per side or until bread is toasted & cheese is melted. Serve warm.

DINNER: Paleo Beef Bolognese Sauce (vegan, low carb)

Prep Time: 10 mins
Cook Time: 30 mins

Ingredients: 1 lb. ground beef, 1 onion (chopped), 3 cloves garlic (minced), 1 carrot (grated), 1/2 tsp.

salt, 1/4 tsp. black pepper, 1 (28 oz) can crushed tomatoes, 1 (6 oz) can tomato paste, 2 tbsp honey, 2 tbsp balsamic vinegar, 1/4 tsp. dried oregano, 1/4 tsp. dried thyme, 1 bay leaf.

Preparation:

-In a large pot over medium-high heat, cook beef, onion, garlic & carrot until beef is browned. Stir in salt & pepper then add crushed tomatoes, tomato paste, honey, balsamic vinegar, oregano, thyme & bay leaf. Bring to a boil then reduce heat to low & simmer for about 30 minutes or until sauce has thickened. Remove from heat then discard bay leaf. Serve over cooked pasta, zucchini noodles, or spaghetti squash.

DAY 83

BREAKFAST: Mediterranean Chopped Grilled Chicken Salad in Romaine Lettuce Cups (with feta cheese)

Prep Time: 10 mins
Cook Time: 10 mins

Ingredients: 1 lb. chicken breast (sliced), 1 tbsp olive oil, 1/2 tsp. garlic powder, salt & pepper to taste, 1/4 cup Kalamata olives (chopped), 1/4 cup sun-dried tomatoes (chopped), 1/4 cup feta cheese (crumbled), 2 tbsp fresh basil leaves (chopped).

Preparation:

-In a small bowl, mix olive oil, garlic powder, salt & pepper.
Brush chicken with the mixture then grill for about 5-7 minutes per side or until cooked through.
Remove from grill then let cool before chopping into bite-size pieces.
Mix together chopped chicken, olives, sun-dried tomatoes, feta cheese & basil leaves in a large bowl.
Serve in romaine lettuce cups.

LUNCH: Low Carb Grilled Veggie Pizza from Shrinking Jeans Kitchen

Prep Time: 10 mins
Cook Time: 10 mins

Ingredients: 1/2 head cauliflower (grated), 1 egg (beaten), 1/4 cup Parmesan cheese (grated), 1 tsp. Italian seasoning, salt & pepper to taste, 1 zucchini (sliced), 1 yellow squash (sliced), 1 red pepper (sliced), 1/4 cup pizza sauce, 1/2 cup mozzarella cheese (shredded).

Preparation:

-In a large bowl, mix cauliflower, egg, Parmesan cheese, Italian seasoning & salt & pepper. Press mixture onto a greased foil-lined baking sheet. Bake at 400 degrees for about 8 minutes then remove from oven. Top with zucchini, yellow squash, red pepper, pizza sauce & mozzarella cheese. Place back in the oven & bake for an additional 8-10 minutes or until cheese is melted. Cut into slices & serve warm.

DINNER: Balsamic Vegetable Stir-fry with Quinoa Pasta or Brown Rice

Prep Time: 10 mins
Cook Time: 10 mins

Ingredients: 1 tbsp olive oil, 1 onion (chopped), 3 cloves garlic (minced), 1 zucchini (sliced), 1 yellow squash (sliced), 1 red pepper (sliced), salt & pepper to taste, 2 tbsp balsamic vinegar, 1/4 cup chicken broth, 1/4 tsp. dried oregano, 1/4 tsp. dried thyme, cooked quinoa pasta or brown rice.

Preparation:

-In a large skillet over medium-high heat sauté onion & garlic in olive oil until softened.
Stir in zucchini, yellow squash, red pepper & salt & pepper.
Sauté for about 5 minutes or until vegetables are slightly tender. Stir in balsamic vinegar, chicken broth, oregano & thyme. Cook for an additional 2-3 minutes then remove from heat. Serve over cooked quinoa pasta or brown rice.

DAY 84

BREAKFAST: Spicy Three-Bean Chili over cooked rice (with cilantro and avocado)

Prep Time: 10 mins
Cook Time: 30 mins

Ingredients: 1 lb. lean ground beef, 1 onion (chopped), 3 cloves garlic (minced), 1 green pepper (chopped), 1 tsp. chili powder, 1 tsp. cumin, salt & pepper to taste, 2 cans black beans (drained & rinsed), 1 can kidney beans (drained & rinsed), 1 can pinto beans (drained & rinsed), 1 (14.5 oz) can diced tomatoes, 1/2 cup tomato sauce, 1/2 cup chicken broth, cooked rice, fresh cilantro leaves, avocado (sliced).

Preparation:

-In a large pot over medium-high heat, cook ground beef, onion, garlic & green pepper until beef is browned. Stir in chili powder, cumin & salt & pepper. Stir in black beans, kidney beans, pinto beans, diced tomatoes with their juice, tomato sauce & chicken broth. Bring to a boil then reduce heat to low & simmer for about 30 minutes or until slightly thickened. Serve chili over cooked rice then top with fresh cilantro leaves & avocado slices.

LUNCH: **Sweet Potato Fries with Spicy Honey Mustard Sauce**

Prep Time: 10 mins
Cook Time: 20 mins

Ingredients: 2 large sweet potatoes (peeled & cut into fries), 1 tbsp olive oil, salt & pepper to taste, 1/4 cup Dijon mustard, 2 tbsp honey, 1 tsp. chili powder.

Preparation:

-Preheat oven to 400 degrees. Toss sweet potato fries with olive oil & salt & pepper. Spread out on a baking sheet in a single layer then bake for about 20 minutes or until golden brown & crispy. Meanwhile, mix Dijon mustard, honey & chili powder in a small bowl. Serve sweet potato fries with the Spicy Honey Mustard Sauce for dipping.

DINNER: **Crispy Brussels Sprouts with Bacon and Pineapple over a Bed of Arugula with Chipotle Lime Mayonnaise & Sesame Seeds**

Prep Time: 10 mins
Cook Time: 20 mins

Ingredients: 1 lb. Brussels sprouts (trimmed & halved), 6 slices bacon (chopped), 1/2 cup pineapple chunks, salt & pepper to taste, 2 tbsp sesame seeds, 1/4 cup mayonnaise, 1 chipotle pepper in adobo sauce (minced), juice of 1 lime, arugula leaves.

Preparation:

-Preheat oven to 400 degrees. Toss Brussels sprouts with bacon, pineapple chunks, salt & pepper. Spread out on a baking sheet & roast for about 20 minutes or until crispy. Sprinkle with sesame seeds. In a small bowl mix together mayonnaise, chipotle pepper & lime juice. Serve Brussels sprouts over a bed of arugula leaves with the Chipotle Lime Mayonnaise on the side.

DAY 85

BREAKFAST: Quinoa Vegetable Chili

Prep Time: 10 mins
Cook Time: 30 mins

Ingredients: 1 lb. lean ground beef, 1 onion (chopped), 3 cloves garlic (minced), 1 green pepper (chopped), 1 tsp. chili powder, 1 tsp. cumin, salt & pepper to taste, 2 cans black beans (drained & rinsed), 1 can kidney beans (drained & rinsed), 1 can pinto beans (drained & rinsed), 1 (14.5 oz) can diced tomatoes, 1/2 cup tomato sauce, 1/2 cup chicken broth, cooked quinoa, fresh cilantro leaves, avocado (sliced).

Preparation:

-In a large pot over medium-high heat, cook ground beef, onion, garlic & green pepper until beef is browned. Stir in chili powder, cumin & salt & pepper. Stir in black beans, kidney beans, pinto beans, diced tomatoes with their juice, tomato sauce & chicken broth. Bring to a boil then reduce heat to low & simmer for about 30 minutes or until slightly thickened. Serve chili over cooked quinoa, then top with fresh cilantro leaves & avocado slices.

LUNCH: Grilled Chicken Caesar Salad over Creamy Lemon Chicken Wrap with Romaine Lettuce

Prep Time: 10 mins
Cook Time: 10 mins

Ingredients: 2 chicken breasts (skinless, boneless), 1/2 head romaine lettuce (chopped), 4 oz shredded mozzarella cheese, 2 tbsp Caesar dressing, 1/4 cup mayonnaise, juice of 1 lemon, 8 small whole wheat tortillas, salt & pepper to taste.

Preparation:

-Sprinkle chicken breasts with salt & pepper then grill (or cook in a skillet) over medium-high heat for about 10 minutes or until cooked through. Mix together chopped romaine lettuce, mozzarella cheese, Caesar dressing, mayonnaise & lemon juice in a large bowl. Lay out each tortilla then top with the chicken Caesar salad mixture. Roll up each tortilla then cut in half.

DINNER: Paleo Cauliflower & Leek Soup with Crumbled Bacon on top with a piece of Whole Wheat Toasted Bread

Prep Time: 10 mins
Cook Time: 25 mins

Ingredients: 1 head cauliflower (chopped), 2 leeks (sliced), 3 cloves garlic (minced), 4 cups chicken broth, 1/4 cup heavy cream, salt & pepper to taste, 6 strips bacon (cooked & crumbled), fresh parsley leaves.

Preparation:

-In a large pot over medium heat cook cauliflower, leeks & garlic in chicken broth for about 25 minutes or until tender.
Purée soup with an immersion blender then stir in heavy cream. Season with salt & pepper to taste. Serve soup topped with crumbled bacon & fresh parsley leaves. Enjoy with a piece of whole wheat toasted bread on the side.

DAY 86

BREAKFAST: Sausage, Egg & Cheese Biscuit

Prep Time: 5 mins
Cook Time: 10 mins

Ingredients: 1 package pre-made biscuit dough, 4 eggs, 8 oz breakfast sausage (cooked), 4 slices American cheese.

Preparation:

 -Preheat oven to 375 degrees. Press biscuit dough into 4 circles on a baking sheet. Crack an egg into the center of each biscuit, then top with cooked sausage & a slice of cheese. Bake in preheated oven for 10-12 minutes or until biscuits are golden brown & eggs are cooked to your liking.

LUNCH: Garden Salad with Grilled Chicken

Prep Time: 5 mins
Cook Time: 10 mins

Ingredients: 1 chicken breast (skinless, boneless), 1/2 head iceberg lettuce (chopped), 1/2 red onion (sliced), 1/2 cucumber (sliced), 2 tbsp Italian dressing, salt & pepper to taste.

Preparation:

-Sprinkle chicken breast with salt & pepper then grill (or cook in a skillet) over medium-high heat for about 10 minutes or until cooked through. Mix together chopped iceberg lettuce, red onion, cucumber & Italian dressing in a large bowl. Top salad with grilled chicken then season with salt & pepper to taste.

DINNER: Spaghetti with Homemade Tomato Sauce & Garlic Bread

Prep Time: 10 mins
Cook Time: 20 mins

Ingredients: 1/2-pound ground beef, 1 small onion (chopped), 3 cloves garlic (minced), 1 (28 oz) can crushed tomatoes, 1/2 tsp sugar, 1/4 tsp dried basil, 1/4 tsp dried oregano, salt & pepper to taste, cooked spaghetti noodles, garlic bread.

Preparation:

-In a large pot over medium heat, cook ground beef, onion & garlic until beef is browned. Stir in crushed tomatoes, sugar, basil, oregano & salt & pepper to taste. Simmer for about 20 minutes or until sauce has thickened. Serve over cooked spaghetti noodles with garlic bread on the side.

DAY 87

BREAKFAST: Scrambled Eggs with Sautéed Spinach & Toast

Prep Time: 5 mins
Cook Time: 10 mins

Ingredients: 4 eggs, 2 cups spinach (chopped), 1/4 cup milk, salt & pepper to taste, 1 tbsp butter, 2 slices whole wheat bread (toasted).

Preparation:

-In a large bowl whisk together eggs, milk, salt & pepper. In a large skillet over medium heat, cook spinach in butter until wilted then add in the egg mixture. Scramble until eggs are cooked to your liking, then serve with toast on the side.

LUNCH: Turkey Sandwich on a Whole Wheat English Muffin with Carrot Sticks

Prep Time: 5 mins
Cook Time: 5 mins
Ingredients: 2 slices turkey breast, 1 slice Swiss cheese, 1 whole wheat English muffin (toasted), Dijon mustard, 1 carrot (cut into sticks).

Preparation:

-Place the turkey and cheese on the English muffin then spread with Dijon mustard. Place the English muffin under the broiler for a minute or two until cheese is melted. Serve with carrot sticks on the side.

DINNER: Salmon with Roasted Asparagus & Sweet Potato Wedges

Prep Time: 10 mins
Cook Time: 20 mins

Ingredients: 1 lb. salmon, 1 lb. asparagus (trimmed), 2 sweet potatoes (cut into wedges), olive oil, salt & pepper to taste.

Preparation:

-Preheat oven to 400 degrees. Toss asparagus and sweet potatoes with olive oil, salt & pepper, then spread out on a baking sheet. Roast for about 20 minutes or until tender. Place the salmon on top of the vegetables, then drizzle with a little more olive oil. Roast for 10-12 minutes or until the salmon is cooked.

DAY 88

BREAKFAST: Grilled Salmon in a Spicy Cilantro Lime Glaze served over Cucumber Noodles

Prep Time: 10 mins
Cook Time: 10 mins

Ingredients: 1 lb. salmon, 1/4 cup cilantro (chopped), juice of 1 lime, 1 tbsp honey, 1 tsp Sriracha sauce, salt & pepper to taste, 2 cucumbers (spiralized into noodles).

Preparation:

-In a small bowl whisk together cilantro, lime juice, honey, Sriracha sauce, salt & pepper. Place the salmon in the mixture then marinate for at least 10 minutes. Preheat grill to medium heat then grill the salmon for about 5-7 minutes per side or until cooked through. Serve over cucumber noodles.

LUNCH: **Walnut Crusted Meatloaf with Cranberry Orange Sauce and Steamed Broccoli**

Prep Time: 15 mins
Cook Time: 1 hour

Ingredients: 1 lb. ground beef, 1/2 cup bread crumbs, 1/4 cup milk, 1 egg, 1 onion (chopped), salt & pepper to taste, 1/2 cup walnuts (chopped), 1/2 cup cranberry sauce, 1/4 cup orange juice.

Preparation:

-In a large bowl, mix ground beef, bread crumbs, milk, egg, onion, salt & pepper. Shape into a loaf then spread the walnuts on top. Bake meatloaf at 350 degrees for about an hour or until cooked through. In a small saucepan, heat cranberry sauce, orange juice, salt & pepper. Serve meatloaf with cranberry orange sauce and steamed broccoli on the side.

DINNER: **Lemon Pepper Cod Fish over Quinoa with Roasted Brussels Sprouts**

Prep Time: 10 mins
Cook Time: 20 mins

Ingredients: 1 lb. cod fish, 1 lemon (juiced), 1 tsp lemon pepper seasoning, 1 tbsp olive oil, 1 cup quinoa, 2 cups Brussels sprouts (trimmed), salt & pepper to taste.

Preparation:

-Preheat oven to 400 degrees. Mix lemon juice, lemon pepper seasoning, and olive oil in a small bowl. Place the cod in the mixture then marinate for at least 10 minutes. Spread the quinoa in an even layer on a baking sheet then top with Brussels sprouts. Drizzle with a little bit of the lemon pepper mixture then season with salt & pepper. Roast for about 20 minutes or until the fish is cooked through and the quinoa is crispy.

DAY 89

BREAKFAST: Chicken with Greens, Feta and Pecans over Couscous

Prep Time: 10 mins
Cook Time: 20 mins

Ingredients: 1 lb. chicken breast (cut into cubes), 1 tbsp olive oil, salt & pepper to taste, 1 bunch greens (chopped), 1/2 cup feta cheese, 1/2 cup pecans (chopped), 1 cup couscous.

Preparation:
-In a large pan, heat olive oil over medium-high heat. Add the chicken then season with salt & pepper. Cook for about 10 minutes or until browned. Add the greens and cook for an additional 5 minutes or until wilted. Stir in the feta cheese and pecans then remove from heat. Cook the couscous according to package instructions. Serve chicken mixture over couscous.

LUNCH: Easy Green Chili Shrimp Tacos

Prep Time: 10 mins
Cook Time: 10 mins

Ingredients: 1 lb. shrimp (peeled & deveined), 1 tbsp olive oil, salt & pepper to taste, 1/2 cup green chili salsa, 8 small soft tacos.

Preparation:
-In a large pan, heat olive oil over medium high heat. Add the shrimp then season with salt & pepper. Cook for about 2-3 minutes per side or until shrimp is pink and slightly charred. Remove from heat then stir in the green chili salsa. Serve shrimp mixture in soft tacos.

DINNER: Paleo Lamb Curry (vegan, low carb)

Prep Time: 15 mins
Cook Time: 30 mins

Ingredients: 1 lb. lamb (cubed), 1 tbsp olive oil, salt & pepper to taste, 1 onion (chopped), 3 cloves garlic (minced), 1 tbsp curry powder, 1 can full fat coconut milk, 1 head cauliflower (chopped into florets), 1 cup green beans.

Preparation:

-In a large pan, heat olive oil over medium-high heat. Add the lamb then season with salt & pepper. Cook for about 5 minutes or until browned. Add the onion, garlic and curry powder. Cook for an additional minute then stir in the coconut milk. Bring mixture to a simmer then add the cauliflower and green beans. Simmer for about 15-20 minutes or until vegetables are cooked to your preference. Season with additional salt & pepper if needed. Serve curry over steamed rice or cauliflower rice.

DAY 90

BREAKFAST: **Banana Oatmeal Pancakes (vegan, gluten free)**

Prep Time: 10 mins
Cook Time: 15 mins

Ingredients: 1 ripe banana, 1 cup rolled oats, 1 tbsp flaxseed meal, 1 tsp baking powder, 1/4 tsp salt, 1 cup almond milk.

Preparation:
-In a blender or food processor, combine all the ingredients and blend until smooth. Heat a large pan over medium heat, then coat with nonstick cooking spray. Scoop 1/4 cup batter for each pancake into the pan. Cook for about 2 minutes per side or until golden brown. Serve pancakes with fresh fruit and maple syrup.

LUNCH: **Spicy Black Bean Soup**

Prep Time: 10 mins
Cook Time: 30 mins

Ingredients: 1 tbsp olive oil, 1 onion (chopped), 3 cloves garlic (minced), 1 jalapeno (seeded & minced), 1 tsp cumin, 2 cans black beans (drained & rinsed), 4 cups chicken or vegetable broth, salt & pepper to taste, 1/2 cup cilantro (chopped).

Preparation:
-In a large pot, heat olive oil over medium high heat. Add the onion, garlic and jalapeno. Cook for about 5 minutes or until softened. Stir in the cumin, then add the black beans and chicken broth. Bring mixture to a boil, then reduce heat to low and simmer for about 20 minutes. Season with salt & pepper to taste, then stir in the cilantro. Serve soup with sour cream, cheese and/or tortilla chips.

DINNER: **Crockpot Chicken Teriyaki (paleo, whole 30)**

Prep Time: 10 mins
Cook Time: 4 hours

Ingredients: 1 lb. chicken breast (cubed), 1/2 cup coconut aminos, 1/4 cup honey, 3 cloves garlic (minced), 1 inch ginger (grated), salt & pepper to taste.

Preparation:

-In a small bowl, whisk together the coconut aminos, honey, garlic and ginger. Season the chicken with salt & pepper then place in a crockpot. Pour the sauce over the chicken then stir to coat. Cook on low for 4 hours or until chicken is cooked through. Serve chicken over steamed rice or cauliflower rice.

DAY 91

BREAKFAST: **Lentil and Rice Soup with tomatoes, carrots and zucchini**

Prep Time: 10 mins
Cook Time: 30 mins

Ingredients: 1 tbsp olive oil, 1 onion (chopped), 3 cloves garlic (minced), 1 cup rice, 1 can diced tomatoes, 4 cups vegetable broth, 1 cup lentils, 2 carrots (chopped), 1 zucchini (chopped), salt & pepper to taste.

Preparation:

-In a large pot, heat olive oil over medium high heat. Add the onion and garlic, then cook for about 5 minutes or until softened. Stir in the rice then add the tomatoes and vegetable broth. Bring mixture to a boil, then stir in the lentils, carrots and zucchini. Simmer for about 20 minutes or until rice is cooked through. Season with salt & pepper to taste. Serve soup with crusty bread or rolls.

LUNCH: **Philly Cheesesteak Burgers on Romaine Lettuce. With Creamy Cheese Sauce & Steamed Broccoli**

Prep Time: 10 mins
Cook Time: 15 mins

Ingredients: 1 lb. ground beef, 1/2 onion (chopped), 1/2 green pepper (chopped), salt & pepper to taste, 1/2 cup shredded cheese, 4 slices cheese, 2 tbsp butter, 2 heads romaine lettuce. For the sauce:

1/4 cup sour cream, 1/4 cup mayonnaise, 1 tsp Worcestershire sauce, 1 clove garlic (minced), salt & pepper to taste.

Preparation:
-In a large skillet over medium-high heat, cook the ground beef until browned. Drain fat then stir in the onion and green pepper. Season with salt & pepper then cook for about 5 minutes or until softened. Stir in the shredded cheese, then remove from heat. Preheat grill to medium high heat.
-To make the sauce: In a small bowl whisk together all of the ingredients. Season with salt & pepper to taste. -Butter one side of each slice of cheese then place on top of burgers. Grill for about 2 minutes per side or until cheese is melted and bubbly. Serve burgers on romaine lettuce with creamy cheese sauce and steamed broccoli.

DINNER: **Paleo Buffalo Burgers (vegan, low carb)**

Prep Time: 10 mins
Cook Time: 15 mins

Ingredients: 1 lb ground beef, 1/2 cup buffalo sauce, 1/4 cup ranch dressing, 1/4 cup bread crumbs, 1 egg, salt & pepper to taste.

Preparation:
-In a large bowl mix together all of the ingredients. Season with salt & pepper to taste then form into burgers. Grill or cook in a skillet over medium high heat for about 5 minutes per side or until cooked through. Serve burgers on buns with your favorite toppings.

DAY 92

BREAKFAST: **Creamy Portobello Mushroom Leek Soup**

Prep Time: 10 mins
Cook Time: 30 mins

Ingredients: 1 tbsp olive oil, 2 leeks (sliced), 4 cloves garlic (minced), 6 portobello mushrooms (chopped), 3 cups vegetable broth, 1/2 cup heavy cream, salt & pepper to taste.

Preparation:
-In a large pot, heat olive oil over medium high heat. Add the leeks and garlic, then cook for about 5 minutes or until softened. Stir in the mushrooms, then add the vegetable broth. Bring mixture to a boil

then simmer for about 20 minutes or until mushrooms are tender. Stir in the heavy cream then season with salt & pepper to taste. Serve soup with crusty bread or rolls.

LUNCH: **BBQ Turkey Burgers topped with Bacon and Cheese over Romaine Lettuce in a Pita Pocket**

Prep Time: 10 mins
Cook Time: 15 mins

Ingredients: 1 lb. ground turkey, 1/4 cup BBQ sauce, 1/4 cup bread crumbs, 1 egg, salt & pepper to taste, 4 slices cheese, 4 slices bacon.

Preparation:

-In a large bowl mix together all of the ingredients. Season with salt & pepper then form into burgers. Grill or cook in a skillet over medium high heat for about 5 minutes per side or until cooked through. Top burgers with cheese then bacon and serve on a bed of romaine lettuce in a pita pocket.

DINNER: **Paleo Chicken Parmesan with Sweet Potato Gnocchi**

Prep Time: 10 mins
Cook Time: 30 mins

Ingredients: 1 lb. chicken breast (cut into tenders), 1/2 cup almond flour, 1/4 cup Parmesan cheese, 1 tsp garlic powder, salt & pepper to taste, 1 egg (beaten), 1 jar (24 oz) marinara sauce, 1 bag (16 oz) sweet potato gnocchi.

Preparation:

-Preheat oven to 400 degrees. Mix the almond flour, Parmesan cheese, garlic powder, salt & pepper in a shallow bowl. Place chicken tenders in the mixture then coat evenly. In a separate bowl beat the egg, then dip chicken in it.
-Place chicken on a greased baking sheet, then bake for about 25 minutes or until golden brown and cooked through.
-Meanwhile, prepare sweet potato gnocchi according to package instructions.
-Serve chicken Parmesan over sweet potato gnocchi with marinara sauce.

DAY 93

BREAKFAST: Grilled Cheese on English Muffin Sandwiches topped with Peppers & Bacon

Prep Time: 5 mins
Cook Time: 10 mins

Ingredients: 4 English muffins, 8 slices cheese, 1/4 cup butter (softened), 1/2 red pepper (sliced), 1/2 green pepper (sliced), 8 slices bacon (cooked).

Preparation:
-Butter the outside of each English muffin then place 4 slices of cheese on 4 of the muffins. Top with peppers, then bacon, then remaining cheese. Place under a broiler or in a toaster oven on low until cheese is melted and bubbly. Top with remaining English muffins then serve.

LUNCH: Bacon Turkey & Brie Omelets with Pineapple Strawberry Salsa

Prep Time: 10 mins
Cook Time: 10 mins

Ingredients: 6 eggs, 1/4 cup milk, 1/2 tsp salt, 1/4 tsp pepper, 1/4 lb. bacon (cooked & crumbled), 1/4 lb. turkey (cooked & diced), 1/2 cup brie cheese (diced), 1/2 pineapple (chopped), 1-pint strawberries (chopped).

Preparation:
-In a bowl whisk together eggs, milk, salt & pepper.
-In a separate bowl mix bacon, turkey, brie cheese, pineapple, strawberries & eggs.
-Heat a large skillet over medium heat, then spray with cooking spray. Pour in egg mixture, then cook for about 2 minutes or until edges start to set. Using a spatula push the edges of the omelet towards the center then tilt the pan so the uncooked eggs flow into the empty spaces. Cook for about 2 more minutes or until desired doneness is reached.
-Fold omelet in half then place on a plate. Serve with Pineapple Strawberry Salsa.

DINNER: Paleo Beef Bolognese Sauce (vegan, low carb)

Prep Time: 10 mins
Cook Time: 30 mins

Ingredients: 1 lb. ground beef, 1 onion (chopped), 3 cloves garlic (minced), 1 carrot (chopped), 1 celery stalk (chopped), 1/2 tsp salt, 1/4 tsp pepper, 1 can (28 oz) crushed tomatoes, 1/2 cup beef broth, 1 bay leaf, 1/4 tsp oregano, 1/4 tsp thyme.

Preparation:

-In a large pot or Dutch oven over medium heat, cook the beef until browned then drain any excess fat.

-Stir in the onions, garlic, carrot, celery, salt & pepper then cook for about 5 minutes or until veggies are softened.

-Stir in the crushed tomatoes, beef broth, bay leaf, oregano & thyme then bring to a boil. Reduce heat to low then simmer for about 30 minutes or until sauce has thickened.

-Remove bay leaf then serve sauce over cooked pasta, zucchini noodles or spaghetti squash. Enjoy!

DAY 94

BREAKFAST: **Stuffed Peppers over Pasta with Tomato Sauce**

Prep Time: 10 mins
Cook Time: 30 mins

Ingredients: 4 bell peppers (halved & seeded), 1/2 lb. ground beef, 1/2 cup uncooked rice, 1 can (15 oz) tomato sauce, 1 tsp Italian seasoning, 1/4 tsp salt, 1/4 tsp pepper, 1 cup shredded mozzarella cheese.

Preparation:

-Preheat oven to 350 degrees F.

-Cook rice according to package instructions, then set aside.

-In a large skillet over medium heat, cook the beef until browned then drain any excess fat.

-Stir in the cooked rice, tomato sauce, Italian seasoning, salt & pepper, then cook for about 5 minutes or until heated through.

-Spoon the beef mixture into the peppers, then place in a baking dish. Pour 1/2 cup of water into the dish, then cover with foil.

-Bake for about 25 minutes or until peppers are tender. Remove from oven then top with mozzarella cheese. Place back in the oven & bake for about 5 more minutes or until cheese is melted.

-Serve immediately. Enjoy!

LUNCH: **Salmon Cakes over Brown Rice with Baby Arugula and Dill Pickles**

Prep Time: 10 mins
Cook Time: 10 mins

Ingredients: 1 can (14.75 oz) salmon, 2 eggs, 1/4 cup diced onion, 1/4 cup diced celery, 2 tbsp chopped fresh parsley, 1/4 tsp salt, 1/8 tsp pepper, 1/4 cup gluten free bread crumbs, 1 tbsp olive oil, 1 cup baby arugula, 4 dill pickles.

Preparation:
-In a large bowl, mix together salmon, eggs, onion, celery, parsley, salt & pepper.
-Form mixture into small patties, then coat in bread crumbs.
-In a large skillet over medium heat cook salmon cakes in olive oil for about 5 minutes per side or until golden brown.
-Serve over brown rice with baby arugula and dill pickles. Enjoy!

DAY 95

BREAKFAST: **Cheesy Quinoa Veggie Burgers with Avocado (vegan & gluten free)**

Prep Time: 10 mins
Cook Time: 20 mins

Ingredients: 1/2 cup uncooked quinoa, 1/2 cup finely chopped bell pepper, 1/2 cup finely chopped onion, 3 cloves minced garlic, 2 tbsp olive oil, 2 tbsp lemon juice, large egg white, salt & pepper to taste.

Preparation:
-In a small saucepan, combine quinoa and 2 cups of water. Bring to a boil then reduce heat to low and simmer for about 15-20 minutes or until liquid is absorbed. Set aside. In a large mixing bowl, combine bell pepper, onion and garlic then set aside. In a microwave safe bowl, heat olive oil, then whisk in egg white, salt & pepper to taste until mixture is frothy. Pour egg white mixture into the bell pepper and onion mixture and mix well. Form into patties and fry for about 5-7 mins on each side or until golden brown.
-In a medium sized skillet over medium heat, add lemon juice and rice burgers to coat in juice. Cook for about 3-5 mins on each side or until golden brown. Serve with sliced avocado and side salad. Enjoy!

LUNCH: Roasted Halibut with Broccoli & Asparagus Sauce with whole wheat couscous or quinoa-based pilaf (vegan & gluten free)

Prep Time: 15 mins
Cook Time: 25 mins

Ingredients: 1 pound halibut fillet, olive oil, salt & pepper to taste, 1 small bunch of asparagus (cut into 1-inch chunks), 2 cups broccoli florets, 1/2 cup diced onion. 1 tbsp ghee or coconut oil if needed.

Preparation:
-Preheat oven to 425 degrees F. Line a baking sheet with parchment paper and place fish on top, then coat in olive oil, salt & pepper and place in the oven for about 15-20 minutes or until fish is cooked through and flakes with a fork. While fish is cooking, place asparagus in a large skillet over medium heat along with 1/2 cup water. Cover skillet and steam for about 5-7 mins then add broccoli florets and onion. Cover and cook for another 5 minutes or until asparagus is tender & broccoli is bright green.
-Scoop out fish from the bones and place in a large mixing bowl. Pour cooked vegetables over top then serve with whole wheat couscous or quinoa-based pilaf. Enjoy!

DINNER: Paleo Chicken & Vegetable Soup with Zucchini Noodles (vegan & gluten free)

Prep Time: 10 mins
Cook Time: 20 mins

Ingredients: 1 tbsp coconut oil, 1/2 large onion, 1 cup sliced carrots, 2 cups sliced button mushrooms, 3 cloves minced garlic, zucchini noodles, 4 cups chicken broth.

Preparation:
-In a large saucepan over medium heat, melt coconut oil, then saute onion, carrots, mushrooms and garlic until soft. About 6-8 mins. Add chicken broth and bring to a boil. Reduce to a simmer for about 20 minutes or until soup is slightly thickened. Serve with zucchini noodles. Enjoy!

DAY 96

BREAKFAST: Grilled Chicken BLT Sliders on Soft Buns

Prep Time: 10 mins
Cook Time: 15 mins

Ingredients: 2 chicken breasts, 4 slices of bacon, 1/4 cup diced sweet yellow onion, 1/4 cup chopped fresh cilantro, 4 slices thick cut bacon.

Preparation:

-Preheat grill to medium high heat. Place chicken breast on the grill then cook for about 10-12 minutes or until cooked through and juices run clear. Allow the chicken to cool, then shred it into small pieces. In a large mixing bowl combine shredded chicken, diced onions, cilantro and seasoning (salt & pepper). -Place slices of bacon across the bottom of the buns, then top with shredded chicken mixture. Top with remaining slices of bacon. Enjoy!

LUNCH: Tilapia in Parchment Paper baked in the oven (baked fish fillets with chopped veggies)

Prep Time: 10 mins
Cook Time: 20 mins

Ingredients: 1 tilapia filet, 2 panko bread crumbs, salt & pepper to taste, 1/2 medium red onion, 3 cups sliced carrots, 3 cups broccoli florets, 1/2 cup diced cucumber, 1 tbsp olive oil if needed.

Preparation:
-Preheat oven to 400 degrees F. Line two baking sheets with parchment paper and keep one extra piece of parchment paper to use later to line the baking sheet again. Place tilapia on the first piece of parchment paper, then season with salt & pepper and press bread crumbs into the tilapia fillet. Place vegetables in a medium sized mixing bowl, drizzle with olive oil and season with salt & pepper then mix well. Spread vegetable mixture onto another piece of parchment paper, place another tilapia fillet on top, then wrap both pieces up tightly with the parchment paper, leaving no openings in the middle. Place on the baking sheet in the oven for about 20-25 minutes or until fish flakes easily with a fork. Remove from oven and allow to cool slightly before carefully unwrapping.
-Carefully unwrap and slice into serving size pieces or as desired then enjoy!

DINNER: Paleo Macaroni and Cheese with Asparagus, Red Onions and Fresh Sage Leaves.

Prep Time: 10 mins
Cook Time: 25 mins

Ingredients: 3 cups macaroni noodles, 2 tsp olive oil, 1/2 cup lemon juice, 1/8 cup diced onion, 4 cloves minced garlic, 4 eggs, 6 cups vegetable broth (plus extra if needed), pinch of salt & pepper to taste.

Preparation:

-In a large saucepan over medium heat, add olive oil, then sprinkle onion, garlic and seasoning. Sauté for about 5 mins or until garlic is slightly browned.
Add in vegetable broth, lemon juice and macaroni noodles. Bring to a boil then simmer for about 15-20 minutes or until liquid is absorbed. Set aside. In a large mixing bowl combine red onions and asparagus then set aside. In a microwave safe bowl, gently heat olive oil, then whisk in egg white, salt & pepper to taste until mixture is bubbly. In a large skillet over medium heat, cook egg mixture for about 6-8 mins or until done. Use a spatula to slice off the edges of the egg mixture and make little flat sandwiches with each piece of egg. Add each piece of egg to a bowl, top with red onions and asparagus then top with cheese.
Enjoy!

DAY 97

BREAKFAST: White Corn & Black Bean Scramble

Prep Time: 10 mins
Cook Time: 15 mins

Ingredients: 2 tbsp coconut oil, 1/2 cup chopped onions, 1/4 cup diced red pepper, 2 eggs, 1/4 cup frozen corn, 1/4 cup black beans.

Preparation:

-In a large skillet, melt coconut oil over medium heat, then toss in onion and red pepper. Cook until soft then add in corn and beans. Cook for about 5 minutes then gently pour the egg mixture into the skillet. As the eggs start to cook, gently push the egg around so that it cooks on top of itself, creating little pockets of scrambled eggs.

LUNCH: Petite Filet Mignon & Sweet Potatoes with Pear Salad

Prep Time: 10 mins
Cook Time: 15 mins

Preparation: 1 lb. petite filet mignon, 4 large sweet potatoes, 1/4 cup olive oil, salt & pepper to taste, 1/4 cup dried cranberries (optional), 2 tbsp chopped fresh parsley.

Preparation:
-Preheat oven to 400 degrees F. Cut sweet potatoes into wedges then place in a medium sized mixing bowl. Drizzle with olive oil, season with salt & pepper then toss well. Place on a baking sheet and bake for about 15-20 minutes or until soft enough to easily pierce. Allow fries to cool slightly then slice into serving size pieces.
-Heat olive oil in a large skillet over medium heat, then add both sides of the filet mignon equally. Season with seasoned salt & pepper, cook for about 5 mins per side or until meat reaches desired temperature (careful due to bone). Allow meat to sit for about 5 mins before slicing into 1" thick slices. Remove from pan and place on a baking sheet. Top with sweet potato wedges, dried cranberries, parsley & seasoning then broil for about 2-3 mins or until heated through.

DINNER: Tandoori Chicken over Basmati Rice & Mango Salad

Prep Time: 10 mins
Cook Time: 15 mins

Ingredients: 1 tsp vegetable oil, 2 chicken breasts, 2 tbsp red curry paste, 1 cup diced onion, salt & pepper to taste.

Preparation:
-In a large mixing bowl, mix red curry paste, salt & pepper then set aside. -Heat vegetable oil in a large skillet over medium heat, add onion, and cook for about 5 minutes. Add in chicken breasts then spread the red curry paste mixture evenly over the chicken breasts until completely coated. Add chopped onion to the middle of the skillet and cover with lid for about 8-10 mins or until chicken is cooked through and juices run clear. Allow to cool slightly before slicing into strips then serve over basmati rice with a side of mango salad.

DAY 98

BREAKFAST: Buckwheat Pancakes & Creamy Avocado Sauce

Prep Time: 10 mins
Cook Time: 15 mins

Ingredients: 3/4 cup buckwheat flour, 1/4 cup coconut flour, 1/4 cup finely diced onion, 2 eggs, 1 1/2 cups almond milk (or preferred milk), salt & pepper to taste.

Preparation:
-In a blender, add avocado, lemon juice, and salt & pepper to taste, then blend until smooth. Add a bit of water if needed just to reach desired consistency. Serve warm or cold.
-In a large mixing bowl, combine buckwheat flour, coconut flour, salt & pepper then mix well. Set aside. In a small saucepan over medium heat, add in almond milk and onion and cook for about 5 minutes or until very little liquid remains. Remove from heat then set aside to cool. In a large mixing bowl, combine coconut flour, buckwheat flour and eggs then mix well. Add almond milk mixture and mix well until batter is smooth. Heat either a nonstick skillet or griddle over medium heat, then pour batter by 1/3 cup full, cook for about 2-3 minutes or until bubbles form on the top of the pancake, then flip. Cook for an additional 1-2 mins or until done. Repeat with remaining batter. -Serve pancakes topped with creamy avocado sauce and any other desired toppings if desired.

LUNCH: Turkey Meatball "Lasagna" in Pita Bread with Romaine Lettuce, Tomato and Basil

Prep Time: 10 mins
Cook Time: 10 mins

Ingredients: 12 oz turkey meatballs, 1/2 cup marinara sauce, 5 oz chopped romaine lettuce, 1/4 cup sliced tomatoes, 2 tbsp basil.
Preparation:
-In a large skillet over medium heat cook meatballs on each side for about 4-5 mins or until cooked through. Set aside then top with marinara sauce and slice half of a tomato. Serve in pita bread alongside lettuce, tomato and basil.

DINNER: Swiss Chard Gratin with Cheddar Cheese, Garlic & Dill and Broccoli Rice

Prep Time: 10 mins
Cook Time: 25 mins

Ingredients: 2 tbsp olive oil, 1/4 cup chopped onions, 2 cloves minced garlic, salt & pepper to taste, 1 tsp dried basil, 1 lb. broccoli florets, 1 cup shredded cheese (any type), 4 cups shredded Swiss chard (1/4 lb.), 1 cup grated Cheddar cheese (any type).

Preparation:

-Preheat oven to 425 degrees F. Grease a casserole dish -Heat olive oil in a large skillet over medium heat then add in chopped onion, salt, pepper and garlic. Cook for about 5 minutes or until soft. Add in broccoli florets and cook for about 3-4 minutes or until soft (do not cook all the way). Remove from heat then mix in Swiss chard, basil & Cheddar cheese.   -Pour into greased casserole dish, then top with shredded cheese. Bake for about 15-20 mins or until bubbly. Remove from oven and serve immediately.

DAY 99

BREAKFAST: **Avocado Blueberry Overnight Oats & Cucumber Mint Salad**

Prep Time: 5 mins
Cook Time: 12hrs

Ingredients: 1 cup rolled oats, 1/.4 cup dried blueberries, 2 tbsp chia seeds, 1 tsp lemon juice, 1/4 cup plain Greek yogurt (optional), 1 large ripe avocado, 3/4 cup almond milk (or preferred milk substitution), pinch of salt.

Preparation:

-Mix non-dairy milk, rolled oats, chia seeds and lemon juice in a pint size mason jar. Add in pinch of salt then close container & shake well. -Place in fridge for about 8-12 hrs. -In the morning, mix all ingredients in a bowl then top with your choice of dried fruit. -Serve over whole wheat toast or other grain of choice with desired toppings/ garnishments.

LUNCH: **Lentil & Kale Burgers with Roasted Carrots, Tomato Raita and Brown Rice**

Prep Time: 10 mins
Cook Time: 20 mins

Ingredients: 1 cup red lentils, 2 tbsp chopped onions, 1/4 tsp cinnamon, 1 clove minced garlic, 2 cups shredded kale (about 2 bunches), 2 large carrots cut into bite-size pieces, salt & pepper to taste.

Preparation:

-In a large skillet over medium heat, cook lentils for at least 10 mins or until soft but not mushy, then add in onion, salt & pepper. Stir well and allow to cook for about 3 minutes or until onions are translucent.
Add in garlic and cook for another minute or until fragrant. Add in carrots then mix well. Allow to cook an additional 3-5 mins then remove from heat and allow to cool slightly. Preheat oven to 425 degrees F. Use a large mixing bowl to gently add in lentil mixture, kale and cinnamon. Mix well, then form into 4 patties and place on a baking sheet lined with parchment paper.
-Bake for 25 mins or until desired done. Remove from oven and allow to cool for about 5 mins before serving. Serve over brown rice with tomato raita.

DINNER: **Pork Teriyaki Lettuce Wraps with Sesame Broccoli**

Prep Time: 5 mins
Cook Time: 10 mins

Ingredients: 1 tbsp olive oil, 2 cloves minced garlic, 2 cups broccoli florets, 3 oz sliced cooked pork, 1 tbsp low sodium soy sauce, 1/4 tsp ground ginger, 1 large romaine lettuce leaf, 1 tsp sesame seeds.

Preparation:

-Heat olive oil in a large skillet over medium heat, then add in garlic and cook for 1 minute or until fragrant.
-Add in broccoli florets and pork then mix well.
-Cover skillet then cook for 3-5 mins or until broccoli is desired crisp-tender, stirring occasionally. -Add in soy sauce, ginger and sesame seeds, then stir well. Serve in lettuce leaf with desired sides.

DAY 100

BREAKFAST: **Homemade Energy Bites**

Prep Time: 5 mins
Cook Time: 12hrs

Ingredients: 2 cups old fashioned oats, 1 cup peanut. butter, 1/4 cup chia seeds, 1 tsp vanilla extract, 2 tbsp honey.

Preparation:

-In a large mixing bowl mix all ingredients by hand or using a whisk until well blended. -Form into desired shapes and place on baking sheet lined with parchment paper. -Place in fridge for about 8-12 hrs. Remove from fridge & let sit at room temperature for 10 mins before serving. -Store covered in fridge for up to 1 week.

LUNCH: **Shrimp & Broccoli over Brown Rice**

Prep Time: 10 mins
Cook Time: 20 mins

Ingredients: 1 tbsp olive oil, 1/2 lb. large shrimp, 1/4 teaspoon salt, 2 cups broccoli florets, 4 cups steamed brown rice, low sodium alfredo sauce (or substitute any other sauce of your choice).

Preparation:

-Heat olive oil in a skillet over medium heat, then add shrimp and salt. Cook for about 6-8 mins or until pink and firm. Remove from heat and set aside to cool. -In same skillet cook broccoli florets & brown rice for about 7-10 mins or until done. Season with salt & spoon Alfredo sauce on top before serving. Serve over brown rice.

DINNER: **Spinach Raviolis with Roasted Butternut Squash, Garlic & Almonds**

Prep Time: 10 mins
Cook Time: 25 mins

Ingredients: 2 large butternut squash peeled, 1 tsp olive oil, 1/2 lb spinach, 1/4 tsp salt, 4 oz ground turkey, 2 cloves minced garlic, 1 tbsp pesto (optional).

Preparation:

-Place squash skin side down on a baking sheet lined with parchment paper and drizzle with olive oil. Bake at 425 degrees F for 25-30 mins or until desired tenderness. -While squash is baking, place a large skillet over medium heat and cook ground turkey for about 4-6 minutes or until browned. Add in garlic and spinach, stir well then cover. Cook for about 5 mins or until spinach is wilted, stirring occasionally. Add in salt & pesto (if using). -In the last 2 mins of squash baking time, fill a large pot with water then bring to a boil. Once boiling add in raviolis & cook for 5 mins or just until tender. Preheat oven to 375 degrees F. Spread pesto on top of cooked squash, then top with ground turkey mixture and almonds. -Bake in the oven for 30-35 mins or until most of the liquid has been absorbed. Serve with desired sides.

CONCLUSION

The book is a great way to jumpstart your journey to a healthier lifestyle. With 300 American recipes, you're sure to find something that fits your taste. And with the morning exercises routine, you'll get your day started on the right foot and make yourself feel more energetic and motivated. No matter what kind of lifestyle you live, there is always room for improvement. Take your health and energy levels seriously, and make sure you learn from the mistakes of others.

This book is a great way to start eating healthy, even if it's just one meal or snack a day. You'll become more aware of what foods are healthy and which aren't, without feeling deprived or like you're missing out on something. This can even lead to you becoming a healthier eater. The trick is to make changes that you can stick with. Start with small steps and start eating better today. You'll be glad you did and your body will thank you.